Reconstructing Identity After Brain Injury

T0383574

Reconstructing Identity After Brain Injury tells the remarkable story of Stijn Geerinck and his journey from road traffic accident to recovery. After he was hit by a drunk driver whilst cycling, Stijn suffered a traumatic brain injury and had to undergo drastic maxillofacial and neurosurgery.

In his own words, this book narrates Stijn's difficult recovery, focusing on the physical, medical, mental, social and financial changes he had to endure. It lays the groundwork for coping with permanent impairment resulting from TBI, including lifelong lesions and the irreversible physical changes. The testimonial narrative is complemented with philosophical insights, providing key philosopher's reflections on the experience of brain injury. Stijn also explores the essential human characteristics of resilience, fighting spirit, emotionality, despair, vulnerability, hope, depression, optimism, anxiety, rationality, focus, anger and love, as he looks at the impact of his brain injury and resulting disfigurement on his masculine identity.

It is essential reading for any professional involved in neuropsychological rehabilitation, and all those touched by this condition.

Stijn Geerinck is a Belgian philosophy teacher, bass player, long-distance runner, and now writer. In 2019 he published his debut book, in Dutch, entitled *Tussen hoop en hersenletsel* (*Between hope and brain injury*). It is an organic narrative about coping with severe bad luck. This work has now been translated in English and its scientific approach aims to support people in similar situations. The author seeks to support wellbeing throughout the world by means of effective altruism, demonstrating how to overcome hardship and disability as far as possible.

After Brain Injury: Survivor Stories
Series Editor: Barbara A. Wilson

This new series of books is aimed at those who have suffered a brain injury, and their families and carers. Each book focuses on a different condition, such as face blindness, amnesia and neglect, or diagnosis, such as encephalitis and locked-in syndrome, resulting from brain injury. Readers will learn about life before the brain injury, the early days of diagnosis, the effects of the brain injury, the process of rehabilitation, and life now. Alongside this personal perspective, professional commentary is also provided by a specialist in neuropsychological rehabilitation, making the books relevant for professionals working in rehabilitation such as psychologists, speech and language therapists, occupational therapists, social workers and rehabilitation doctors. They will also appeal to clinical psychology trainees and undergraduate and graduate students in neuropsychology, rehabilitation science, and related courses who value the case study approach.

With this series, we also hope to help expand awareness of brain injury and its consequences. The World Health Organization has recently acknowledged the need to raise the profile of mental health issues (with the WHO Mental Health Action Plan 2013-20) and we believe there needs to be a similar focus on psychological, neurological and behavioural issues caused by brain disorder, and a deeper understanding of the importance of rehabilitation support. Giving a voice to these survivors of brain injury is a step in the right direction.

Published titles:

The Reality of Brain Injury
Am I Still Me?
Andrew Tillyard

For more information about this series, please visit: https://www.routledge.com/After-Brain-Injury-Survivor-Stories/book-series/ABI

Reconstructing Identity After Brain Injury

A Search for Hope and Optimism After Maxillofacial and Neurosurgery

Stijn Geerinck

Routledge
Taylor & Francis Group
LONDON AND NEW YORK

Cover image: Michel Goessens

First published 2022
by Routledge
4 Park Square, Milton Park, Abingdon, Oxon OX14 4RN

and by Routledge
605 Third Avenue, New York, NY 10158

Routledge is an imprint of the Taylor & Francis Group, an informa business

Translated by Thomas K. D. Mermans

British Library Cataloguing-in-Publication Data
A catalogue record for this book is available from the British Library

Library of Congress Cataloging-in-Publication Data
A catalog record has been requested for this book

ISBN: 978-1-032-07054-4 (hbk)
ISBN: 978-1-032-03649-6 (pbk)
ISBN: 978-1-003-20514-2 (ebk)

DOI: 10.4324/9781003205142

Typeset in Times New Roman
by Taylor & Francis Books

Contents

Figure

About the Book

This book documents a search in extreme conditions, the winding road from relapse to recovery of a road traffic victim. Stijn Geerinck was hit by a drunk driver while cycling and had to undergo drastic maxillofacial and neurosurgery at Ghent University Hospital (Belgium). This story narrates the various aspects of his arduous recovery (physical, medical, mental, social, financial, …) and lays the groundwork for a method to cope with permanent impairment resulting from acquired brain injury (ABI), lifelong lesions and the irreversible change in his body and particularly his face… Although the story itself is in no way generalisable and every ABI comes with different degrees of quality of life, it is nonetheless an attempt to illustrate an often-stated though also an often-underestimated truth: that life can be worth living, even in circumstances that on the surface seem to imply otherwise. Insights from philosophy and philosophy of science complement this testimonial narrative.

Preface: Life, Survival and Personal Identity

One morning, I ran into Stijn Geerinck on the basement floor of Ghent University Hospital – the campus I'm working at. He recognised me as his former teacher and started talking to me. I, however, hardly recognised him: he had become a different person. He briefly explained that a drunk driver had run into him and that he had barely made it out alive, that he had had multiple surgeries (among which the removal of his bone flap) and that there had been a lot of complications, that the accident had changed him for the rest of his life.

To this day, I can remember the conversation very vividly, especially how even though the accident had ruined a significant part of Stijn's life, he didn't have any negative things to say. He talked about the bone flap removal as if he were talking about lifting a casserole lid to see if its contents were done yet. Stijn was still in recovery but clearly remained hopeful and determined to get back on his feet again.

And then we were both on our way, he to the next step in his recovery and I to an interview, followed by a lecture I had to teach. It was unreal. I was truly touched and moved by that conversation and still am to this day. How can one find the courage and hope to carry on after so much misery? What does this mean for one's identity? What impact did it have on those around them?

Someone I knew was also a road traffic victim with an acquired brain injury (ABI), so by now I had a somewhat better understanding of what it entailed. Still, empathy is but a theoretical consideration and can only do so much: it does not allow one to actually take someone else's place. What did they, their family and friends go through? What was it like to have to recover time and time again?

Stijn provides an answer to those questions in this book. He takes us with him on his long and arduous journey to recovery and does not leave out any of the challenges he faced. Throughout this personal story, the reader will encounter philosophical questions about identity, the impact of technology on our body and appearance, as well as the most important of all questions: what is the meaning of life? Why do we fight for our survival? What makes us willing to invest so much courage and energy into carrying on? This and many other questions are discussed in this courageous testimony.

Stijn is not alone. I would like to quote French philosopher Jean-Luc Nancy, a man also confronted with a life-changing medical journey. Nancy had had a heart transplant and suffered from cancer in its aftermath. In his touching description of its impact, he writes:

> I am both open and closed. In between lies an opening through which strangeness is pouring in incessantly: medication to suppress my immune system, other drugs that combat so-called minor side-effects, but also effects that cannot be combatted (such as the deterioration of my kidneys), frequent examinations … My entire existence, in short, has been put into a new perspective, shaken to its foundations, scanned and reduced to different registers, each with its own possibility of death.[1]

Just like Nancy, Stijn accurately describes the sheer size of the impact that the accident and all interventions it necessitated have had. A medical history leads to alienation from one's former self, but also offers the opportunity to reinvent oneself.

I highly recommend reading this book and hope that it will inspire many people, be it patients, friends and relatives, caregivers or anyone with an interest in the subject of this story.

Prof. Dr. Ignaas Devisch
University of Ghent

Note

1 Nancy, Jean-Luc (2010) *L'Intrus.* Paris: Editions (translated by Thomas K. D. Mermans).

Introduction

This book reports my personal reaction to extreme and life-threatening events. It is my individual exploration of the essential human characteristics of resilience, fighting spirit, emotionality, despair, vulnerability, hope, depression, optimism, anxiety, rationality, focus, love of life and of others, friendship, anger … It is the contribution of an experienced member of the universal working group called 'advanced recovery'.

To put it differently: I hope that people facing challenging and demanding situations will find something useful among the insights and experiences shared in this work. I hope there will be a meaningful outcome to what I went through. I hope to offer support to others and to make a difference, to provide something of value.

This, of course, is not to say that just about anyone in a situation similar to mine can count on the same lucky outcome if they just follow my lead. Although rehabilitation takes a lot of work on the part of the injured person, scientifically, it is known that outcomes are in large part the result of the type, location and extent of the injury sustained and the amount of rehabilitation the person has received. It is not just due to the character or effort of the person with the injury. The all-familiar saying 'if you work hard you can get wherever you want to' is sadly just not true for everyone, as even I have come to find. To say otherwise would not only be scientifically incorrect, but moreover incredibly invalidating to the brave and arduous battle many people fight against overwhelming suffering. My aim is therefore not to divulge the ultimate remedy to all ails, but merely to make a valuable contribution to effective rehab from experience, to show that, in many (though not all) cases, a certain state of mind can go a long way.

This book has been a valuable document to myself and plays an essential role in working on my recovery. I started translating my experiences into words as soon as I was able to and have not stopped since out of sheer relief that it seems to keep on working and that my

DOI: 10.4324/9781003205142-1

consciousness continues to exist. It has also become an attempt to turn the story into something meaningful for a wider audience and society as a whole. It is the beginning of the next chapter in my life. The story is written in the past tense and sometimes features coloured boxes containing thoughts and concepts from podcasts and books I resorted to as soon as I had regained consciousness. It was my way of spending lonely hours of waiting, of overcoming time and life coming to an abrupt halt. They are written in the present tense.

The book was written under conditions of impaired consciousness, which is why it meanders from one subject to another despite the fact that they may have happened simultaneously. This in itself is a testimony to the organic way this work has grown. Repetition and the lack of a strictly chronological development reflect the nature of the story: these were the circumstances in which I tried to introduce a clear and unambiguous structure.

Most people who live through my experience do not survive, or at least, not as the same person. They mostly come out mentally impaired to various degrees or with a personality that has changed tremendously. This was not (or less) the case in my situation, which makes this story unique in and by itself. It documents my exploration of what was still possible during my recovery.

Chapter 1

A Radical Change

The End of a Lucky Duck

I used to be the happy-go-lucky sort of person, the man for whom every day was Sunday both as a child and as an adult. I had a wonderful family, a meaningful job and fantastic hobbies that gave me great joy. I was a father of two children with a lovely wife, a teacher of philosophy in secondary education, a bass player in a groovy band and a long-distance runner. Add to that a group of the finest friends one could wish for and it is fair to say that life was good to me. The fact that all this was set in an affluent region such as Flanders[1] at the beginning of the 21st century undoubtedly contributed to that feeling of prosperity. The world I lived in knew no major problems such as war, poverty or rampant inequality. Of course, it would be an exaggeration to say everything just fell into my lap. Even under the most favourable conditions chances do not take themselves. However, although some days came easier than others, there were no insurmountable obstacles and I was always one to count my blessings.

> Apart from any possible personal merits, my prosperity was mostly a matter of extremely beneficial circumstances. I was no stranger to happy coincidence: it was my faithful ally. My imagination turned 'Every day is like Sunday, every day is silent and grey' into 'Every day is like Sunday, every day is vibrant and gay'.
>
> I don't know Morrissey (the writer of the original soundbite) personally but he has always struck me as a witty and enjoyable representative of a rather gloomy view on life. In my opinion, he shows that seemingly contrasting views of life are not necessarily irreconcilable.

And then I turned 40, a transition that would have been trite and uneventful if it weren't for the life-changing incident that shook my world. It was my first encounter with bad luck, a common fact of life

DOI: 10.4324/9781003205142-2

but in this case nonetheless a blow of massive proportions. I became a traffic accident victim, pure and simple, a split second with drastic consequences. In the blink of an eye, in a jiffy, I was left with a confusing mess of dramatic and far-reaching outcomes. It was the beginning of the greatest challenge of my life.

The accident was the start of what would turn out to be a radical confrontation with my own personality. Willpower and perseverance were put to the test to see whether they were only empty words, hollow theoretical shells, or would actually live up to their name and withstand the hostility of reality. Was my talent for optimism just an unfounded attribute or actually a useful weapon for life? How far did my ability to make life worth living reach, to make a positive difference to those close to me (family, students, friends) even in moments of hardship?

What happened? Spring 2017: as I was riding my bike on a nightly trip, a drunk driver, who had fallen asleep behind the wheel, mercilessly crashed into me. The police were called and the perpetrator would later have to stand trial. I was taken to the nearest clinic, which was Ghent University Hospital, a place that specialised in the sort of care my situation required. It literally saved my life. Their neurosurgeon was (and still is) a star at lonely heights in his line of work. Even though calling the fact a 'lucky break' would be a bit inappropriate given the severity of my situation, it was most certainly a silver lining to a very dark cloud. The fact I was transferred to this hospital very fast is the only reason I survived. I became a statistic, not as a casualty but as a survivor of a traffic accident by merits of medical technology and positive science. I got to see what it means to be human in the Modern Era from up close and in the most radical way. The achievements of our exceptional cognitive abilities were what kept me alive. On the flipside, however, I had become a victim of one of the many disadvantages of modern public infrastructure.

> Public spaces are mostly regarded as functional environments, meant to bring us from one place to another in fast and dangerous vehicles. Within this domain, any contact with others is to be avoided due to its inherent dangers. This leads to human alienation. The person who ran me over apparently no longer considered the road a place where one is to take responsibility towards others. By boxing ourselves in moving cans called cars we have significantly increased the distance between one another. Although most of the available means of transportation are efficient and have massive advantages, one could argue they don't really fit our bodily nature. Neither our senses nor our psychological abilities are adapted to high speeds and a complex interplay of events in the modern functional 'pseudo-open space'.

The challenge was to preserve the connection to what's positive and valuable in life. I reckoned it would become a long struggle. Luckily, I nonetheless felt determined to write a second chapter to my story, one that would be worthwhile.

The accident left me with an acquired brain injury (ABI). For three months, my skull had to stay open after surgery to give room to my severely injured and swollen brain. At the same time, I suffered from the issues that come with 'sinking skin flap syndrome'. The gravity of the situation called for an urgent replacement of my bone flap in spite of a hospital bug I had caught and which made surgery particularly risky. Luckily, I came out without further damage. The next step was to install a permanent shunt to drain any superfluous cerebrospinal fluid, which had been heaping up in my ventricles since I fell out of bed. It was supposed to remain there for the rest of my life. Adjusting the shunt, however, proved to be difficult and initially, too much fluid was being drained. As a result, I had to spend the next couple of weeks lying head-down on an inclined bed. To make things worse, I suffered from double pneumonia. My fall from the bed convinced the medical staff to take no further risks and strap me to the bed every single night for four months.

I had broken my cervical vertebrae column, so it was decided it would be best to stabilise my neck with something called a Halo vest – a metal brace attached from my middle body to the top of my head that was supposed to keep my cervical vertebrae in place. I spent the next three months with this brace around my upper body, with only a 'sheepskin' to support the construction and make things more comfortable – although this proved to be a burden rather than a blessing, especially during summer, as I soon found out. The entire left side of my body was paralysed. My face had taken the worst blows and was severely disfigured, which also had an impact on my heavily injured eyes. The damage was said to be irreversible and situated in the right temporal lobe.

It was impossible to assess the outcome of these events, especially at the early stage of the revalidation process. As I was unable to take in food for a long time, I lost more than 20 kg. My consciousness was too impaired to eat without assistance and I found myself continuously at risk of choking. It was much more likely than not that I would come out a different person and / or severely mentally impaired – if I survived the ordeal at all, that is. I did survive, albeit with many complementary and simultaneous complications. My future perspectives were grim and short-lived.

Neurosurgeon Prof. Dr. Kalala made an important announcement to my parents and my wife: 'Once we've replaced the bone flap, Stijn will be able to reach the same level as right after the incident and to live a life worth living.' This meant a lot, because my situation had only deteriorated the first months after the accident.

The food intake issue was resolved soon after said announcement by continuously having a feeding tube in place, first via the nose and later via the abdomen. Also, I was transferred back to Ghent after a short relocation to Oostende due to the fact that I had 'run out of bed-days',[2] a bureaucratic disaster that all but cost me my life had it not been for the impressive prowess of the nursing staff in Oostende (shout-out to Sabine and her colleagues).

I hold no conscious memories of this time after the accident. Everything I know was told to me by my wife and parents. I hardly spoke a word at the time and it stayed that way until after my skull was reattached and my speech gradually improved. In all, I had to go through the cycle of 'intensive care – high care – hospital – revalidation' three times.

The life that gently drifted on the flow of seemingly unstoppable progress came to an abrupt and irreversible end in a matter of seconds. It was replaced by an existence of insecurity and a dubious future with only one certainty: I would be dependent on others for an indefinite amount of time and unsuited for work for a long while. The intensity and duration of this period was impossible to predict, so I could only hope that whatever form of bodily resilience I possessed would not fail me now. The first weeks I was in mortal danger without conscious thoughts or feelings. I had to undergo my situation passively: the feeble faith in a life-worthy outcome was reserved for the surgeons. My parents, wife and kids were dependent on their assessment and decisions while I spent my time in the waiting room of unconscious existence.

Having stayed by my side for the first three weeks all by herself, my wife decided to bring my two daughters to the intensive care department. My oldest daughter had prepared a speech but couldn't read it out loud. Mom had to read it for her, while we all listened, hand in hand. At the end of the visit, I waved to them, the first sign of demonstrable consciousness, save for the way I had been holding hands with my wife for some days by then. I made contact, I communicated at last.

The accident and the recovery had made one thing painfully clear to me: my mental identity and its bodily vessel, the brain, are one and the same. My conscious experience is rooted in the functioning of my brain. I went into an identity crisis, embarked on a life-long journey in search of new equilibria, driven by the obligation to reinvent myself.

What is commonly considered the essence of humanity was suddenly endangered in an overwhelming fashion. My ideas, memories, convictions, fantasies, emotions, 'tools for thinking', … they were all under threat. I was about to lose myself irrevocably. In the course of many months, I became more and more aware of the complexity of the human brain.

The fact that the human organism is powered by a rich variety of processes has become clear to me through the lens of my 'extreme situation'. Unsurprisingly, there is a multitude of brain-related possibilities and difficulties alike. Listing them all here would simply take too many pages, as my experience soon made me realise. The way I process stimuli has drastically changed, the pieces of my thinking abilities have to be put back together from scratch and I am facing a long, capricious and untrodden trajectory learning how to come to terms with my new reality. It will take most of my energy for a long time.

I had to trust in the remarkable plasticity of the brain for my recovery. A significant area was affected and I could only hope that the neighbouring regions would take over the tasks of the damaged tissue. I had learned from a reliable source that neurons are not like skin or blood cells. Neurons that are destroyed are generally not replaced, so it was up to the survivors to fill the functional gap. I soon came to see the utility of 'brain training' and was constantly trying to stimulate cooperation and healthy competition among the remaining brain cells, relying on the neurotherapy provided by the K7 rehabilitation centre of Ghent University Hospital. I often joked that I had become the rare owner of a brain going through puberty for a second time (although my limited consciousness prevented me from riding the wave of my black humour). It only came to me relatively late in the recovery process, an afterthought in every sense of the word.

Notes

1 The northernmost, Dutch-speaking region of Belgium.
2 The number of days a patient stays overnight at the hospital.

Chapter 2

The Mental Resilience Reflex

Perseverance was key, as was claiming all conscious moments that had become so precious to me. For months, I lived in the well-nigh hermetically sealed bubble of the here and now.

As time progressed, I slowly developed the mental resilience to ward off relapse, the ability to embrace bad luck and the feeling of injustice that comes with it. I called it 'the mental resilience reflex'. It took me months to develop it before I could call it as such during a conversation with my friend Wouter (the drummer of my band). All it took was for him to ask me how I was doing. I had a challenging and busy day ahead of me: seeing my lawyer, a final revalidation session in preparation of the facial reconstruction surgery, having over a film crew shooting a documentary on facial surgery at Ghent University Hospital – a tough combination for an ABI patient. I told him it was hard, but that I 'tried to develop an almost spontaneous reaction to stop apathy or depression from getting the best of me.'

Giving it a name and honing the skill was my way of shaping my willpower. It had to be a more or less spontaneous reaction, a stubborn, powerful and positive reflex to bad luck, fear and physical or mental decline. At times, it proved to be almost impossible, but that only further encouraged me to resort to what had kept me going: my family, running, music, reading, writing, friends, going out and talking, carrying on slowly but surely at a sensible pace … All these things helped me a lot and lie at the heart of the reflex. Although I realised that the form these lights in the darkness take differs from person to person, I nonetheless had the feeling that my mental resilience reflex could have universal value, because it was based on human nature and shaped by natural selection. That basis was (at least in theory, in my opinion) available to all. It became my main objective to develop and learn this ability.

I worked hard to cope with difficult circumstances as rationally as possible. I wanted to see results, whatever it took. This was clearly a

DOI: 10.4324/9781003205142-3

break with my easy-going style before the accident. My mental outlook was thoroughly analysed in an attempt to root out all thoughts and actions that stood in the way of my recovery. For example: I made no allowances for lashing out at other people (although lifeless objects often had to suffer for it). Drinking was too risky and would have conflicted with the principles of recovery, so I stopped completely and indefinitely. Instead, I set strict priorities into which I put all my available energy. I found out that without any theoretical background in cognitive behavioural therapy, I nonetheless had come to similar conclusions and approaches in the course of my rehabilitation.

We often don't have any control over the things that happen to us, but we can choose to some extent how we interpret them and how we feel in response to them. This is hard, but not impossible. Although much also depends on one's character and circumstances, there is an opportunity to exert control over our rational and emotional reaction to reality. This opportunity is limited, but nonetheless real and partly manageable, enough to be significant, in my experience.

The Socratic method[1] also contributed to this insight. I validated the arguments that supported my own views and opinions by having a debate with myself to test my mental framework. I tried to align my approach with the harshness of reality. I already had some professional experience with this through my work as a philosophy teacher working with people with an autism spectrum disorder (ASD) and both normally and highly intellectually gifted youngsters. I renewed and practiced this skill with the help of my wife and children. The result was an exceptional vantage point. I tried to use my new perception of reality to my advantage and to the benefit of those around me.

The basis and starting point of my method is applied philosophy. I often use the Socratic method to source the input for the discussion from the pupils themselves. In my classes, we constitute a sort of research community that tests the value of arguments that underpin our convictions and opinions. Pupils also learn in a safe environment how to react to different opinions. For example: if you hear a statement you don't agree with, don't stop listening, but try to see things from the discussant's perspective and compare his arguments to your own. This will hone your own thinking. To my mind, this is a very valuable skill for life.

One often-used and fruitful tactic was to stimulate the production of serotonin and endorphin through what I called 'glorified long-distance race walking' (I had become really slow), that is to say, jogging within the boundaries imposed by my injuries.

Playing with my kids and talking to my wife were also helpful. Reading and writing my texts or class preparations gave me a lot of energy. By writing, I created stimuli-free circumstances. I shut myself into the text. It was a highly desirable confirmation that I was conscious again and it also allowed me to steer and express my restless mind.

Even watching the chickens in the garden for an hour or so contributed to my positive outlook. I sometimes pictured how the Ancient Greek philosopher Epicurus[2] must have felt in his dearly beloved garden. I was lucky to have so many trees and wild birds close to my home, the realisation of which was often enough to face the challenges of my recovery with renewed vigour. I was looking forward to having my friends over in this open space in what would hopefully be the near future.

An important part of my resilience reflex is the way I summarise my state of mind, both inside my head as well as during conversations with others. I want to tell a positive story. It is a short version of the facts with a focus on what is still possible, away from the permanent aspects of my impairment. I resort to the same phrasing in every encounter, so much that it has become a 'tested expression' (more on 'tested expressions' in the chapter on 'Language against the Impairment'):

> I have managed to preserve my personality, which isn't a small thing for anyone with a serious brain injury. Mentally and cognitively, I'm on the same level as before and I am no longer in a wheelchair. Also, I still have my family, parents and friends around me. The very fact I can have this conversation, that I can express these thoughts consciously is nothing short of a victory. It feels like a huge blessing.

These are all unexpected strokes of luck that truly boost my optimism, but it is hard to express in words the enormous mental struggle that precedes them. It takes daily efforts to keep on believing in the optimistic version of my story myself and it will be this way for the rest of my life. The more I recover, the more overwhelming that experience seems to be. I have to resort to the resilience reflex on a daily basis. My motivation constantly requires renewal and actualisation. To go about my day in an acceptable and purposeful manner takes much more energy than it used to. As a result, I have become very attached to the things that raise my spirits.

I had a lot of therapy to work on (amongst others) my mental resilience throughout my recovery and I had many conversations with Prof. Dr. Engelien Lannoo, a neuropsychologist at Ghent University Hospital. I started to compare it to the support top athletes often get from their coach and their team. I had run a marathon before – albeit a relatively slow one at a speed of 10.5 km/h and in 3 h and 58 min –, so I speak from experience when I say that recovery was harder, more demanding and more complicated. Sometimes, I tried to lift my spirits by telling myself that to run once again for 10 km would be by no means a smaller achievement than to become a world champion of cycling or to finish the Tour de France and make it into the top 10 – a slight exaggeration, yet still a realistic assessment of my predicament. In any case, it helped me to carry on, head and hopes held high.

Ever since the accident, I've been continuously relying on my reflex, 24/7. A relentlessly recurring fatigue and irrational feelings of being pressed for time prove to be particularly persistent. I have developed a compulsive obsession to achieve, to be productive, to make things happen, to complete objectives. It continuously takes all of my conscious energy.

The question remains how much this will change over time. Am I stuck with this insatiable unrest for the rest of my life? Will I be able to also use this aspect of my changing identity to my advantage? Will I find peace and quiet in my head without any mental decline as a result? I reflect on all this in more detail in the section on 'time and desire'.

I realised early on in my recovery that the mental resilience reflex could only work if it was founded on a clear and thorough basis, also on an emotional level. To that end, I used another 'tested expression':

The unconditional, fundamental goal of my reflex is to offer a useful and meaningful perspective on life to my daughters. That's what they deserve and need. Even when life gets hard, there are often still valuable options. This insight is what I want to demonstrate and elaborate.

Notes

1 A conversational technique in which two conversational partners (or, *in casu*, a dialogue with oneself) draw out assumptions underlying a premise by asking critical questions and using them to falsify the argument. Named after its first famous practitioner: Socrates.

2 A Greek philosopher famous for his garden where he and his followers often spent time, seeking reclusion and the simple circumstances they maintained were necessary for happiness (Konstan, 2018).

Reference

Konstan, David (2018) Epicurus, in Zalta, Edward N., *The Stanford Encyclopedia of Philosophy*, https://plato.stanford.edu/archives/sum2018/entries/epicurus/.

Chapter 3

Physical Recovery

In terms of physique, the unfortunate turn of events in my life had given me the feeling that my body had become that of a very elderly man overnight. My entire left side was paralysed, I could not move and had to use a wheelchair, my left arm would not budge … My face had been dealt the heaviest blows, both aesthetically and functionally. Its entire left side was paralysed, I could no longer express myself verbally and was unable to close my left eye or open the right one – in addition to the risk of becoming completely blind or partially sighted. Eating and talking took a tremendous amount of effort, so that I could only have mixed or mashed foods. All dishes consisted of large scoops of food, as if it were ice cream.

For the first time in my life, I felt a burning thirst for revenge, revenge against the accident and its consequences. This became clear when I finally got the opportunity to leave the wheelchair and could use a walker instead. Every free moment between therapy sessions I went to the garden of the centre, got up from my wheelchair and walked around the garden with my walker. All my spare time was used to this end for weeks, under the watchful eye of my therapists. I tried to use my stubbornness and hatred in a positive way and to steer the inevitable sense of frustration away from people towards inanimate objects. The emptiness of my room was often subjected to verbal abuse and I got into the occasional fistfight with a wall or door.

Giving Me a Fighting Chance: Surviving as a Road Traffic Victim

Neurosurgeon Prof. Dr. Jelle Vandersteene had promised my wife the day after the accident that he would do everything in his power to give me a fighting chance. The first days would be crucial and unpredictable. My condition was critical and my prospects uncertain. For at

DOI: 10.4324/9781003205142-4

least three days on end, I was in mortal danger. My family had to wait for 72 hours to see if I would make it or not, after which the chance of death would gradually decrease. My medical resuscitation started with the removal of my bone flap (for three months, as it turned out) and was followed by a multitude of surgical interventions. The determination of the surgeon and the wonders of medical technology ultimately saved my life.

Literally no one expected me to pull through without any severe disabilities. My resuscitation was to be long and uncertain. It's hard to express in words the length of my journey from unconsciousness to full awareness. Even the nursing staff reacted with disbelief to my situation: many had never seen something like this before. My wife could count on a lot of compassion and empathy from those around her, but at the end of the day, the one to make this journey by himself was me.

Thanks to medical progress, many people survive severe road traffic accidents, more than ever before in history, statistically speaking. This is an astounding evolution in itself. My story bears witness to this fact and illustrates the special and fragile way in which survivors re-enter society. I hope I can offer some insights that will facilitate this arduous come-back for others.

For many months, I couldn't live at home, but had to stay at the K7 rehab centre of Ghent Hospital instead. It took me some weeks before I developed a sense of orientation in this foreign place, navigating my wheelchair through unknown corridors. Eventually, I learned that my room was located at the side of the elevator opposite to the therapy rooms – the beginning of a renewed sense of orientation. Within these walls, I gradually regained my spatial awareness. However, there still was the problem of me getting upset by unknown sounds. The noise people produced often seemed like screams of desperation and powerlessness. I hardly understood what they were saying and didn't know where they were coming from. My disturbed ability to process stimuli had a hard time keeping up with all this. It made me feel anxious and agitated in the weeks it took me to adapt to this aspect of the situation. Oftentimes, I felt the urge to help, but I was tied up in bed and simply couldn't do anything. The nurses had their hands full comforting and assisting the many residents of K7.

Every day, my schedule was filled with various forms of therapy: occupational therapy, physical therapy, speech therapy and neurotherapy – truly, I became part of a therapeutic community! The latter was an advanced form of brain training with exercises to improve memory, concentration, searching connections, problem solving, spatial awareness and logical thinking. My results were meticulously registered and compared over time. Together, these were important parameters to eventually determine my level of disability and to see whether I would be suited for work or not. This mattered a great deal to me, as I did all that I could to be able to work again, with the help of An, Sofie and Annelies, my neurotherapists who were very patient and supportive. I wrote down my lesson preparations and filled in the gaps of my existing course material. If I could finish the schedule in time, I would be able to cover the entire mandatory curriculum for the non-confessional ethics course with subjects of my own choosing. I would be able to get back to work well-prepared – a huge relief, given that I would return as a different person to my pupils. My personality might have remained intact, but my circumstances as a teacher had thoroughly changed. This was especially so at the time of the Great Relapse, when I failed to stick to the schedule, thus aggravating the fears and doubts about getting back to work after all the effort I had put into allaying them. Once again, however, neurotherapy and the therapists managed to pull me through it.

Physical therapy was mainly focussed on keeping my balance and learning how to walk. Jolein, Jeroen and other therapists carefully adapted the training to my impairments. After some time, I also started training abs and endurance, especially by swimming increasingly longer distances in the hospital pool, once a week at first, later twice, using my walker to get there.

Speech therapy was an attempt to reactivate my face. I worked my way through an intensive series of pronunciation exercises and tried to develop facial expressions.

My occupational therapists – Jens, Jonas, Astrid and their many colleagues – assisted me in relearning daily activities. At first, I needed help washing and getting dressed and it was not until September 2017 that I could take a shower again – albeit under therapeutic supervision. It was a moment to remember, because I was finally able to trade in my fixed collar for a detachable version. For the first time since the accident, I had the feeling of being fully clean. Later, the principal focus of therapy shifted to learning how to ride a bike, use public transportation and how to safely navigate public spaces. The observation that even 'ordinary' daily activities were no longer easy hit me hard. One time, for instance, when I could use my credit card again, I had forgotten the code, so a new one had to be installed. Even memorising four miserable digits seemed to be too difficult because I had lost my motor skills and my sharp eyesight. I reacted with anger and disappointment. Camille, the physiotherapist who was with me at the time, had to use all her skills to calm me down and called upon the soothing voice of my wife over the phone. It worked, but it seemed to me that the road to 'normality' would be a long path leading nowhere. Anyway, it was clear I needed therapy – a lot. The meaningful work of the therapists at the centre made all the difference to me. Thank you, all of you!

So I resided for three months at the hospital and for six months at the rehab centre. At the end of my stay, I was given the chance to try and live more independently in a 'therapeutic apartment', which was two floors below that of the regular rooms. Funny little detail: this was the only time in my life I was in possession of a spacious wardrobe with automated doors! This phase was the ultimate test to see whether returning home was realistic. I had to cook easy meals without putting myself in danger, to get up in the morning without help and to wash all by myself, so I could make it to therapy in time – in short: an initial step towards normal life. My first attempts brought about quite some stress and consequently the therapists who had to keep an eye on me had their hands full. Progress was slow and irregular, and required all my available willpower.

A Radical but Rational Reaction to the 'Great Relapse': Epilepsy and More

After more than a year of gradual progress and foreseeable relapse, something unexpected happened. The brain damage I had sustained turned out to be so substantial that I had become susceptible to epilepsy. One day, without warning, I went down and landed on my face during what would turn out to be my first epileptic attack. It ushered in a new era of additional sorrow over the stability of my brain, a setback of massive proportions: the 'Great Relapse'. It left a deep impression on me.

The time after the epileptic attack (summer of 2018) saw a true relapse in all aspects of my recovery. All the effort I had put into regaining acceptable cognitive and physical levels for a year was undone in the blink of an eye. In many respects, I had to start all over again. At the very least, there was solace in the fact that the epilepsy was but a mere sign of damage already sustained, so it didn't mean per se that I could expect any further deterioration. Moreover, as I had hoped, it would turn out to be a one-time only surprise as far as the stability of my brains was concerned – a lucky break if you asked me, given the circumstances. Still, this consideration proved to be quite relative. What was directly impacted, for instance, was my short-term memory. The distance between reality and my perception thereof seemed to have increased again. If I went through my schedule for the day and the one after with my wife, I often had to ask up to three times how things were organised. It reminded me of what I had heard about my time in the ICU. My stay there was one big black hole and all I can remember is what I managed to piece together based on the stories of my parents, my wife and my children. My first weeks at the rehabilitation centre too had become a grey area. All in all, many months of my conscious life had gone to waste.

To make matters worse, I received yet another blow in the same week as my epileptic attack. The ear doctor had discovered that further scarification of my left ear and the resulting decrease in hearing meant that my left ear would never function again. The epilepsy and permanent hearing loss were the first impairments without any hope of recovery and as such threatened to completely destroy my hope of making progress. My goals seemed so distant, I was stopped in my tracks on the road to normality and slowly began to drift away from its destination. My recovery was on the verge of total collapse due to yet another stroke of bad luck.

I became more and more aware of my increasing vulnerability. When I was rehearsing with my band, for example, I almost sustained hearing loss in the only functional ear I had left. Ever since the accident, I had used ear plugs while practising. I was well aware that damage to my right ear would mean the irrevocable end of my life as I knew it. I would become deaf or hard-of-hearing and thus be unable to teach anymore, I would have to give up my hobby as a musician – a true doom scenario, especially after my previous ordeal. That fateful night, I had removed the plugs when the playing was over. Suddenly, the sound installation emitted an unexpected, ear-deafening bang, caused by the sound settings of the laptop that was connected to it. I feared the worst but got off with a fright.

My recovery up to that point had taught me much about overcoming hurdles. Still, the 'Great Relapse' felt like a new beginning. In spite of its similarities with previous experiences, there now was something different: the setback was drastic, overwhelming and, especially, unexpected. I had never foreseen such a substantial relapse. It confronted me in a harsh, unfiltered way with the vulnerability of my situation. Of course, we are all vulnerable in our own way, as my wife rightly pointed out, but I had the feeling that this had exponentially become the case for me, disproportionally so to what I could still take.

Would this simply be too much for my mental resilience, the blow of adversity that would do me in, the straw to break the camel's back, the final resistance crushed by harsh reality? I had a strong feeling it would be indeed. When I finally fully realised this, I decided that only a radical reaction could fight the relapse and preserve the positive attitude that had amply proven its worth in the past but was now facing a seemingly insurmountable problem. It was time for some decisive action.

I decided to re-enrol for sports therapy, effective immediately, after a break necessitated by the epileptic attack. I knew all too well from previous experience the direct neurological impact of physical exercise and wanted to maximally exploit its wholesome effects. Swimming at least 1 km twice a week in the nearest Olympic-size pool became a top priority, as did a slow form of long-distance running. The goal was to get back to 10 km while gradually increasing the speed.

A realistic approach of my new objectives was paramount if I wanted to succeed. I went about it well-prepared. To exert control over all possible aspects, I used my heart rate monitor and GPS more intensively than ever before. I made sure to stay well within the limits of my physical abilities by rationally analysing my level and carefully monitoring my speed. I kept it low enough so I could keep up the pace, only increasing it to improve my condition for the sake of recovery, no longer to break personal records. I started out exceptionally slow and only marginally increased the speed. Long-distance running turned out to be the most workable discipline for my condition. I made a path by treading it, race-walking it out of nothing.

Long-distance Running and the Precedent of the Marathon

My choice to become a long-distance runner had always been one of the best and happiest I had ever made. Back in 2016, I had been fortunate enough to run the 'In Flanders Fields' marathon in Ypres and was preparing for a second one at the time of the accident. It proved to be a game changer for my recovery. Virtually all the bones of my sternum had been broken by the collision, as had been my neck, right beneath the skull. Nevertheless, none of these fractures had resulted in displacement, thanks to, amongst others, the muscles I had built that kept it all in place, thus saving me from severe paralysis and the inability to turn my head. Of course, credit also goes to the decision made by Ghent Hospital not to permanently fix my neck with a metal implant but to use a Halo vest instead. All in all, I made it out of my wheelchair fairly quickly. Also, I realised that rationality is key for my recovery from my marathon preparations. By always staying well within my limits during training, I managed to avoid injury and make slow and incremental progress.

During the previous marathon in Ypres, I fell for the classic mistake of hubris. After 33 km, I felt so great that I decided to step up the pace significantly, though I hadn't trained for it. My body reacted poorly and retaliated with severe muscle fatigue. The final 8 to 9 km were hell and I crossed the finishing line in tears.

After the accident, I realised that, from now on, I couldn't afford such a mistake. My increased vulnerability would simply not allow my body to recover sufficiently. It motivated me to systematically act rationally, to move boundaries without being irresponsible about it. It was an exercise in balance, the refinement of a pragmatic but decisive approach.

Evolutionarily speaking, it makes perfect sense that our body is so well-suited to walk and run. For millions of years, we continuously migrated to find food. Natural selection gave rise to a body adapted to this form of existence and movement, allowing us to cover long distances at a relatively slow pace. What we are not made for, by contrast, is to sit still in a chair in poorly ventilated spaces. We were built for bridging large distances. Muscles and joints, however, still have to get used to it. Evolution doesn't follow a perfectly delineated plan. The unpredictability of a continuously changing environment has had a huge influence on the changes in our body, for better and for worse. A good understanding thereof helps to make well-advised decisions. To train wisely is key.

What works well for me is to start by gradually increasing the distance. Once a particular goal has been achieved (5, 10, 15 km), I slowly step up the pace, before once again focusing on distances. During my recovery, I even started to no longer care about speed, by necessity and the will to get my priorities straight. Most of all, I wanted to keep on running, both because I enjoyed it and because it is one of the best ways to maintain my condition. To be in decent shape is essential for achieving significant physical and mental goals, and that's exactly what I want.

I had had the pleasure of discovering the source of energy that is long-distance running before the accident. Like many others, I had faced mentally challenging periods before and isolated

them through running, thus making them manageable. After the accident, I was determined to do it all over again, like never before.

A moment to remember: the first time I succeeded at going from speed-walking to jogging. I was still staying at the rehab centre when my physiotherapist suggested I ran a little in the corridor – slowly, of course. I had spent several weeks trying to take some strained steps, at first with my walker and later without. Better still, after a couple of months, I had managed to get up from my wheelchair and walk through the corridor and garden of K7 every day since. Now, as unbelievable as it seemed, I even ran for the first time. Up until then, I had never thought it possible. Words cannot adequately describe the way I felt that day.

Seven months after the accident, it got even better. In an attempt to raise my spirits after a mentally challenging start of the day, my wife and daughters (nine and eleven years old) took me for a run around the pond at the recreational site of Blaarmeersen in Ghent. This was not without risk for my confidence. That family outing was to show the exact measure of my impairment and I would make it or break it, and fortunately, it turned out to be a true success. Although it was a shock to see I couldn't keep up with my children despite their young age, the joy I felt sharing this moment with my family left no room for disappointment. I managed to complete a whole lap, a triumph of about 3 km, with the three 'women of my life'. I was overcome by an indescribable feeling of joy. In that instant, my approximation of normal life became more tangible than ever before. It had been a long and difficult journey, but I was back. Dad was standing on his own two feet again, running a lap all by himself.

About nine months after the accident, I got back to 10 km, albeit more as a form of 'glorified speed-walking' than actual running. I was incredibly slow, but I pulled it off, gradually stepping up the pace. However, the epileptic attack about three months later set me back tremendously and I went from 7.5 min/km to about 9 to 11 min/km, which is, as experienced runners can confirm, incredibly slow. Even the distance I could cover was reduced to a mere 3 km. The fact I was still able to run at all was the only straw to grasp at. Running had been my shelter from negative feelings. To see it slip away like this was incredibly difficult. I felt the anger boiling inside of me and it was hard not to give up altogether. The only time I had been this slow was when I had first stood up from my wheelchair. It felt like all these months of struggle had been in vain. It was up to running to save me again.

I decided to combine running with two weekly swimming sessions at the rehab centre's pool again. For a couple of months, I swam about an hour or so and covered 40 lengths of 25 m at first and 55 lengths later on, before I was discharged and had to continue at the Olympic pool of Rozenbroeken at Ghent. It was an opportunity for me and my family to rediscover the joy of family activities. We had a blast. Swimming, running and family time – an important combination for someone in recovery.

I often resorted to my background in sports and counted my lucky stars for having run that marathon at Ypres. Time and time again, I went looking for that mysterious rhythm of the body only experienced in endurance runs. That rhythm became a symbol of my gritty reaction against the impairment. It had always been the closest thing I knew to spiritual feelings. My mind, though usually mostly concerned with reason, was no stranger to the 'runner's high'. My current circumstances added extra spice, an extra dimension to that experience and symbolically opened the door to a steady recovery.

A month after the 'Great Relapse', I went back to 10 very slow kilometres, by some sort of 'glorified speed-walking' (it had become a tested expression) rather than by running. The feelings that came with it are hard to describe, but let's say they were not unlike the satisfaction of sweet revenge.

All this was made possible only by a thorough, rational approach of the situation. I consistently kept well within my limits (especially when it came to pace) to prevent further injury to my already injured body and to gain more energy from the endeavour than it cost me. Day after day, I adhered to strict discipline and worked on well-defined objectives. I was determined to create the perfect blend of the fruits of medical progress (of which I was the beneficiary, neurologically speaking) and those of my self-developed willpower. I would overcome. And so, I started running, leaving in my wake the accident, the epileptic attack, urethroplasty, facial surgery, the financial problems ...

Hooray for repetition, I did it again! Though it must be said: the power of repetition is very much underestimated. I owe this insight to Prof. Hugo Van Den Enden, one of the best teachers I ever had. My recovery illustrates this well. Repetition was one of the reasons I made more progress than anyone had dared to hope for.

(Also to successful organisations, repetition is gold. To rely on the same old well-defined routines may sound boring, but it is essential for order and structure. The same goes for difficult pedagogical challenges, where addressing the heart of the problem again and again with patience, understanding and clear boundaries can often go a long way.)

Long-distance running reconciled my rational disposition with the (universal human?) need for spirituality. The latter had always been something I wasn't very receptive to. When I say spirituality, I don't mean religion. It was the secretion of chemical compounds such as dopamine and serotonin while running that made me feel connected with the chemical composition of the cosmos. Knowledge of the building blocks of reality helped me exploit my limited options and apparently, to some extent, I could steer the reactions in my body that governed my mood. This realisation was sufficient to engage me in the reality of my physical surroundings. Running long distances showed me this wasn't merely a theory: it made me feel it, accommodating both my rational and my emotional needs.

It made me wonder whether both sides were truly opposites. They rather seemed complementary.

Both emotions and rationality have a material origin in the brain. This unique combination, these two sides of the same neurological coin have given us an incredible evolutionary edge. And what's most remarkable: since the Cognitive Revolution some 70,000 years ago, when we started to develop language and culture, we have become aware of these competitive strengths, more so than any other species has ever been aware of theirs. This is not quite what you can call the most original conclusion, but nonetheless, it is one that feels authentic and very present in challenging times. It encourages me to continue working on the 'transformation of emotions'.

Endurance running with brain injury clearly led to more profound rational and emotional observations and its value became all the more apparent under these difficult circumstances. It was my instrument to achieve challenging goals during recovery, my very own lesson in accepting pain, exhaustion and the hard confrontation with my limits. But there was more to running than just its contributions to my recovery. Week after week, it showed me what's truly important, it taught me to carefully set the pace in all aspects of life, to care for my environment. It made me believe in a meaningful future again. Life sure hadn't lost its excitement: running was the confirmation that I still loved being alive. Even extreme situations wouldn't stop me from seeing my 'second life' as a gift, despite the mental and physical hardships and limitations. It went to show the true nature of my personality and the strength of my bodily system, much to my relief. Along with the technological revolution, our welfare state and the support of those around me, my character and resilience made me live again.

Thanks to endurance running, I was connected with life's changes again, to that never-ending game of continuous evolution. Running gave structure to my unstoppable thoughts and to my slowly awakening memory. Physical exercise is what woke up my damaged brains.

Increasing distance and speed proved to be difficult and largely dependent on the stage of my recovery. This was especially the case after the facial surgery, probably because I took on a lot. I never bit off more than I could chew, but still, I was willing to take more risks than before. How was I to progress if I didn't know the extent of my limits? I had to seek them out, to see how far I could make it on the road to what life used to be. I had done it before, but then more carefully so and one boundary at a time. Now, I went all-in: my family, my work and hobbies, writing, glorified speed-walking … What had seemed impossible in earlier phases now became achievable, and God knows I made the most of it. I had to fine-tune my energy consumption profile and no obstacle was going to scare me off.

Injured for Life

Although I made it further in recovery than expected, time nonetheless revealed a harsh reality. One year later, it became clear to me I would be injured for life. The experts had always maintained it was well-nigh impossible for someone as injured as I to come out completely intact – for that, the brain injury was simply too great and the collateral damage too extensive. It gradually became clear to me what this truly meant. As it would turn out, my experience would make me an expert in brain-related problems, such as life-long acquired brain injury, defective sensory processing and trouble with resolving unexpected problems.

The daily struggle with fatigue and a diminished load capacity was a given. It became manageable over time, but still: it was always there. Coffee (the only addiction I allowed myself to give in to, apart from chocolate) was my go-to in an attempt to feel more energetic. For a long time, I tried to overcome my sleepiness by going to bed early and limiting my evening activities to a minimum. It didn't help. I lay awake for hours, tired but unable to sleep – a bizarre sensation. It was as if my mind had become so attached to my regained consciousness that it wanted to make the most of every minute. My wife often asked me what worries kept me up at night but worrying simply wasn't an accurate denominator for the issue. Some thoughts, of course, were gloomy in light of my difficult situation, but that wasn't all there was to it. All scenes of my life, both negative and positive, were depicted in an internal show without end. I couldn't stop it. What my mind lacked in short-term memory, it made up for in nightly séances with ghosts past and present, the good kind and the bad.

Partial paralysis of my body prevented me from closing my left eye. This didn't get any better, contrary to my arm and leg. I continuously had to use eye-drops and to apply ointment before going to sleep. My right eye socket was shattered and had been removed, which made my eye sink away into my face. My left ear was beyond the help of even a hearing aid. It had lost its function to a fracture of the petrous part of the temporal bone and to a severely damaged cochlea. They only broke the news to me 14 months after the accident. From now on, I had to make do with my right ear, so I wanted extra protection. I ordered custom earplugs to continue to play music and do my job as a teacher, afraid of losing my hearing entirely.

The damage to my left ear had also affected my balancing organ, again irreparably so. Luckily, the central and right zones of my nervous system turned out to have taken over. Under dark, wet or wintery circumstances, my balance was limited. Driving home by bike in winter, for instance, was simply too dangerous, as was using a ladder without help, trimming trees or cleaning out roof gutters. Still, my sense of balance wasn't completely unresponsive to training and I noticed clear progress thanks to my stubborn attempts to take the stairs with the help of the guardrail and all the speed-walking sessions.

A couple of muscles had been severed in the process of removing my bone flap and a poor blood flow had led to tissue necrosis and the consequent loss of part of my skull. It had left me with a crater at my right temple, which to some extent was corrected by surgery, but was nonetheless still clearly visible afterwards. And then there was my sense of orientation that had become a constant source of uncertainty and stress. I often felt rushed or constantly under unfounded time pressure.

Crossing the Finishing Line of the Medical Trail Run: Facial Surgery

It felt like my face had become the face of another.

It represented the most visible aspect of my impairment and stopped me from speaking, breathing or eating freely. I did recognise myself in the mirror, but it always reminded me of the words of my doctor: 'Sir, you have to accept that your body has changed.' I was forced to behave differently and make different choices in life, and my face was a daily reminder of that.

After a year and four months, they offered me the possibility of undergoing facial surgery. It was a tough choice to make. I had been through many medical interventions, so taking on yet another one wasn't exactly something I was looking forward to. 'Why can't they just leave my body alone?' I often jested sarcastically.

The surgery would take 11 hours under complete anaesthetic. Fat tissue and blood vessels from my own leg would be transplanted to my face, along with a long nerve that would wind up from left to right between my nose and upper lip. After being allowed to grow for nine months, the latter was supposed to reactivate the left half of my paralysed face and the nerve of my left mastication muscle, to which it would be connected. The main objective was to make my mouth work, so I could laugh, talk and eat naturally again. While they were at it, they would also correct my left nostril and take in my unclosable left eye so that it would match its right counterpart. The intervention would on the one hand restore balance and symmetry in my face (what could be called a 'passive aspect' to the endeavour) and on the other breathe life into my facial muscles (an 'active aspect').

This was nothing short of an organisational wonder, executed by both facial and plastic surgeons of Ghent Hospital. Professor Hubert Vermeersch and Professor Phillip Blondeel had pulled off a face transplant eight years before, so I was in good hands, both technically and in terms of the peace of mind they inspired.

Still, it would also be a conscious choice for significant relapse. By now, I knew from experience what that meant, so it became an almost impossible dilemma. Especially the fact that this was the first time I had to make such a conscious decision myself caught me off guard. The previous interventions had been decided for me. I couldn't prepare for this and had to rely on my instinct.

For a long time, I had maintained that I didn't need any merely aesthetical corrections, but as my abilities to eat, breathe and eat were on the line, these qualms weren't really relevant objections. I was unable to pronounce some words correctly, particularly those containing a 'p'. Chewing fluently and keeping food in my mouth was impossible and the air flow through my left nostril was significantly hampered by the paralysis. This was an obstacle, both to my work as a teacher and to daily life. Also, it affected my confidence. Moreover, I looked different, rather 'impaired'. The entire left side of my body was half-paralysed, but it was my face that recovered the least, with all the practical and aesthetical consequences it entailed. Besides children gawking at my face on the tram, there was also the noticeable reservation and suspicion of adults I crossed in the streets.

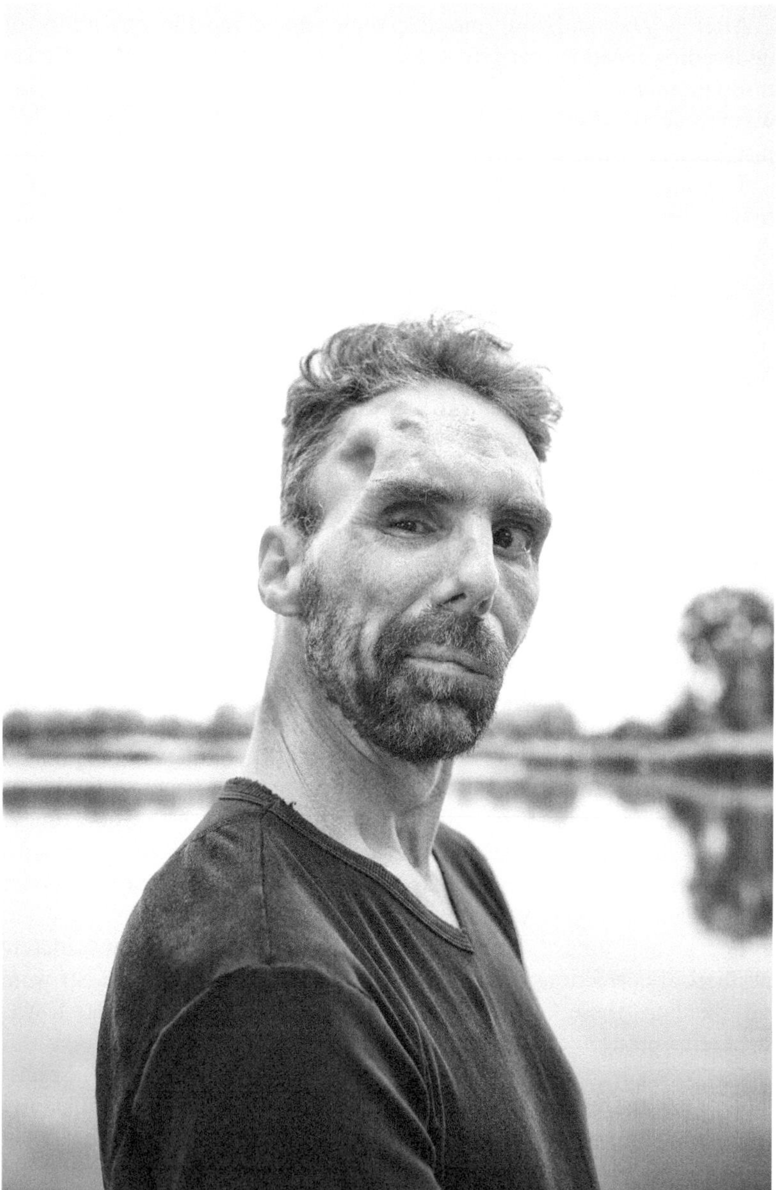

Figure 3.1 Aesthetic impact of the accident on my face
Note: Even after the first round of facial surgery, the results remain significant.

The biggest confrontation with the consequences of my new look came in the first weeks, when I started working as a teacher again, right before the facial surgery. I used the first moments in front of the class to explain the situation to relieve my pupils of their questions and uncertainties. Already pupils I didn't teach had come to me on the playground, uneasily asking what had happened. Usually, they did so with great care as to not hurt my feelings, though there was one youngster who didn't care much for subtleties and referred to me in English as 'the man with the deformed face'. Luckily, I didn't feel offended or hurt, but it sure was a wake-up call. I took solace from my unuttered comeback that soon, he would have to call me 'the man with the reformed face'.

Of course, besides the objective of making life more practical, there also was an aesthetical side to this intervention. Maybe they could throw in some Brad Pitt-like features, or maybe a little bit of Clooney … I came well-prepared with jokes for the occasion.

> Any feeble quips from yours truly – possibly even present in this manuscript – can always be conveniently attributed to my supposedly diminished sense of restraint, caused by the brain injury. The worse the humour, the more relevant it becomes to share it out loud – and get away with it anyway.

It didn't take me long to agree to the surgery. I fought moments of doubt with rational arguments and a firm belief in the reputation and status of the surgeons. It was a hard yet resolute decision.

Nonetheless, I chose to decline part of the proposed alterations. Reconstructing my right eye socket would be a complicated intervention requiring months of preparation (in which even engineers would play a part) and targeting an area close to the brain. This was not without danger, so I decided not to undergo it. Exposing my brain to unnecessary risk was out of the question.

Right after the surgery (September 2018), I felt a remarkable change. The surgeons had said that they would resuscitate my face, and that's exactly how it felt. I recognised myself again. I experienced a restored balance and harmony between what I looked like and who I truly was on the inside. I became deeply aware that a face is more than a superficial billboard for the outside world: it is also the symbolic representation of one's personality.

I worked hard every day to recover the unique aspects of my personality. It was a long exercise in reclaiming my individuality. Like everyone else, I took my place in society by using my personal talents and strengthening them. During the 40 years preceding the accident I had used them to build self-esteem and social status. In this respect also I had to start all over again. I had to establish new foundations. Fortunately, I was mentally and cognitively able to draw in part on old assets.

My face between the accident and the surgery didn't reflect this inner struggle, on the contrary: it gave physical shape to the irreversible aspects of my predicament. It forced those around me to continuously compose themselves and react in a certain way. Some kept their distance, while others reacted with a disproportionate amount of empathy. I noticed lots of averted eyes among acquaintances. I assumed that everyone did the best they could and didn't let it get me down. I had other things on my mind, so wasting too much energy on this was not an option. I did realise, however, that this situation would become psychologically challenging in the long run.

The human face, moreover, plays a central role in establishing initial, spontaneous contact between people. Empathic, altruistic and open-minded communication between strangers or casual acquaintances often starts with face-to-face interaction.

I longed to express empathy again by just looking at someone and showing them my face. I learned from experience the way people instinctively measure up others.

This instinctive assessment often precedes the actual acquaintance, only then rational considerations follow, and even then oftentimes only as a justification of the initial emotional evaluation.

The distrust was palpable. I looked deep into the essence of this reaction, searching for its root cause to understand and accept it.

Evolutionarily speaking, we have always depended heavily on collaboration. To maintain collaboration, we need to single out the cheaters. People often subconsciously engage in predictive cheater-detection, confident in their ability to foresee whether someone is suited to collaborate with or not. For this, they interpret different signs, of which facial expression (besides clothing, behaviour, complexion, ...) is the main one. The danger is therefore that one can jump to conclusions based on false stereotypes and moral prejudice. Many people fall for it and believe they can read trustworthiness and other personality traits in someone's face.

Research shows that people who smile come across as more trustworthy and that a symmetrical smile instils more empathy and trust than an asymmetrical one. One theory has it that a symmetrical smile comes from emotion areas deep in the brain and that people instinctively consider it therefore more spontaneous, and hence more genuine.

People often follow their gut-feeling in their assessment of others – a 'sixth sense' or an instinct, as it were. This, however, is far from a flawless method and there is a limit to the reliability of facial information, in spite of its popular conception as a 'window to the soul'. In the past, it even gave rise to the elaborately described pseudoscience of physiognomy, an ancient discipline based on the conviction that one's personality can be derived from their appearance.

Another important sign of trustworthiness is the look in one's eyes. Children aged one pay much more attention to eye movement than other hominids. If we don't trust our conversational partner, it is useful to study their eyes. This gives us some information with regards to their sincerity. Signs of trust, however, are under heavy evolutionary pressure because of cheaters trying to imitate them. Cheap and easy signals have been filtered out by natural selection so that we are left with signs that are hard to mimic, such as a spontaneous smile or eye contact. Of course, they can be faked, but it is hard to. Therefore, people constantly tend to screen faces (based on Verplaetse (2008)).

I could no longer smile symmetrically, which was a problem in itself. The look in my eyes too was affected by the asymmetry in shape and size due to the partial paralysis of my face and the loss of my right eye socket.

The facial correction freed me from the universal yet understandable restraint at the sight of my disfigured face, the awkward moment of confusion expressed as internal questions such as: 'Can I properly interact with this person to an acceptable degree? Is he mentally able to understand me? How does anyone incur such disfigurement?'

Functionally too, I immediately noticed significant progress. People noticed my speech had become clearer, food could stay longer in my mouth while chewing, breathing through the nose went more smoothly and now happened through both nostrils.

Facial surgery was a crucial, necessary step in a resolute and permanent evolution to normal life. The facial and neurosurgeons of Ghent Hospital have saved my life, both literally and figuratively. Their intervention physically affirmed my mental resilience. I felt strong, despite the discomfort after the surgery. Fortunately, recovery didn't take as long as was the case for the neurosurgical intervention and was limited to one week in hospital. The effect of the anaesthetic was long but superficial.

Already in the first week, I managed to free up some energy for meaningful activities that by now had become part of a well-established rehab tradition. It felt like a big step forward. I wasn't quite back on my feet yet (although I took my first slow steps already on day three), so I decided to read and write – a lot. Luckily, I could count on the understanding and help of my family and parents. Clearly, I was still in good company. Seeing the amount of energy I could free up at this early stage, I got my hopes up for improving my fatigue levels and diminished load capacity. I was already looking forward to getting back to work as a teacher in six weeks.

The first few days, I was almost euphorically optimistic. By the end of the first week, I was nonetheless forced to recognise the gravity of the intervention. My progress in terms of mobility stagnated as quickly as it had begun, fatigue was slowly catching up on me and the long anaesthetic had an undeniable impact.

Recovery had become more familiar through experience, but not necessarily easier. I understood clearly that it would take time and energy and that I had to be patient. Still, the many sorts of relapse throughout my rehabilitation remained enormously challenging mentally, although the realisation that this could very well be the last time things would go steadily downhill offered some comfort. It made me all the more eager to get back to normal for good. But first, I'd have to focus on the challenges in front of me, both big and small.

My old enemy fatigue was back at it again. It had always been there, lurking in the background, but now it really took the stage in the drama that was this relapse. Once again, I had to tread carefully and with thorough deliberation, looking for the boundaries of my abilities and persisting in rational slowness. I had to keep moving, maintaining the balance between rest and exercise.

The surgeons had taken great care to leave my muscles and tendons unharmed while taking materials from my leg. Some degree of recovery, however, was unavoidable. The removal of the nerve made walking challenging and I often had the feeling of stepping into shards of glass with my left foot. It got better by the day, but it was nonetheless a slow evolution. I had to walk extra slowly and avoid abrupt, uncontrolled movements.

During the surgery (which took 11 hours), I had to be tubed through my urethra. Given my urethra's history up until that point, it took special permission from the urologist to go ahead as planned. The week after the surgery, however, I noticed that relieving myself had become more difficult, which made me worry. Still, I had enough of all the unexpected interventions, especially now that I considered myself discharged at last, so I decided to wait and hope for the best. I did the same in the case of my resurfacing blurred vision, which I attributed to fatigue and let be for the time being.

All these setbacks on so many different levels constituted a major hurdle. Once again, I was surrounded by challenges coming in from all sides and adding to the steepness of the way ahead of me.

And then it was over. Finally, after eight serious medical interventions, four of which in life-threatening conditions, I could breathe again in the prospect that this was likely to be the last one. This was the first time I had some sort of outlook on medical retirement.

One month after the surgery, my family and I took our next big step going on a holiday to the Ardennes with Joke and Beorn, another couple we were friends with. We were hoping to make a walking holiday out of it, which was risky in light of my newly regained mobility and the damage to my balancing organ. We decided to take a calculated risk by adapting distance and trajectory to my physical reality. I was determined to once again push my boundaries in a responsible, well-advised way, to start moving again in a challenging yet realistic environment, and for that, the forests of Rochefort were the ideal location. Good company and the gorgeous colours of autumn reaffirmed my desire to live. I was with my wife and children all the time, which allowed me to reclaim my position in our family. I felt like I was back, a great source of motivation that reconnected me with a happy and valuable existence.

The freed-up space in my head, however, was soon taken by new preoccupations. I experienced a change in the way my brain dealt with life. Before the accident, it tended to leave room for emptiness. It didn't take much effort to stop a train of thought and entertain pleasurable ideas about light-hearted subjects. Taking a nap was easy in those days, I was quick to be distracted and never one to worry (with the exception of one personal loss). Now, however, it seemed my mind had become more dynamic and untameable.

At the time, I found myself at a crossroads of various events. I was about to pick up work again for a second time with the intention to do as much as possible. Next, there was my absolute priority: to be there for my wife and kids every single day in a profound and meaningful way, not just for a while, but permanently. I was also finally able to truly restart my social life. Besides practising and performing with my band, I started attending events again, such as de Nacht van de Vrijdenker (the Night of the Freethinker), the Breinwijzer Festival on free will, … all connected with the content of this manuscript. Working on this text and trying to turn it into something worth calling a book was one of my main occupations. I wondered whether my restlessness was caused by the brain injury or by my circumstances. In general, I assumed it was a combination of both factors.

All in all, the dominant feeling was still one of uncertainty and unpredictability. It was impossible to accurately foretell the feasibility of my dreams and ambitions. I came significantly closer to what is generally considered to be daily normality, which made me all the more eager and happy, but at the same time, I was perfectly aware of the fragility of the situation and the continuous, drastic influence of my brain injury. I had good reason to hope for a decisive victory over the impairment – an encouraging thought, but not one to leave room for euphoria in the face of imminent overconfidence. Fortunately, I knew the pitfalls. I couldn't lose track of the pace. I grew impatient about finishing my book and though I enjoyed the process of writing it, I nonetheless was eager to publish and felt inner unrest. I had to refrain from getting ahead of myself. Impatience would have disastrous outcomes.

All these difficulties were typical of this stage of my recovery and, like previous problems, were true challenges for my injured brain. I got the impression that my restless thoughts were here to stay forever – although it did come with certain advantages. In spite of the hecticness, it made me a more motivated thinker, with a bigger aptitude for in-depth exploration and for following a line of thought to its final destination.

I had been in fighting mode for months, and not out of choice. My life had become a life-or-death situation which left no room for reflection or relief. I had learned a healthy form of aggressive focus to cope with reality. Now, after some time, there were finally some moments of rumination. This was a remarkable emotional experience, a sensitive confrontation with the nearly indescribable nature of my very own zero-sum game.

There was a moment, some weeks after the facial surgery, that illustrates this feeling well. I had managed to get tickets for a musical hero of mine, Johnny Marr, in Antwerp. My wife and I attended the show. Different factors led to an emotional outburst of tears. I ran into some old friends I thought I'd never see again and it put my life and its extreme turn for the worse into a different perspective, so when Johnny started playing 'There is a Light that Never Goes Out', I cried like a child. The lyrics, the amazing guitar riff, the memories of before, the sudden awareness of my wounded and fragile presence… it all gave rise to an emotional outburst, and I spontaneously visualised the many scars on my body. It was proof I was still able to cry and I was immediately convinced this was a good thing. In addition to the physical and mental recovery, there now also was an emotional renaissance, another step towards claiming an authentic personality, towards feeling more human.

It was a hard confrontation with reality. I had always been someone who did well in the fast lane, living with eagerness and convinced that I was at the top of my game. I was a busy bee. I constantly commuted back and forth between my work, my family and a busy social life. After the accident, I was forced to distance myself from my previous self. I felt that life was continuously changing and evolving, but instead of standing at the helm, I now had to undergo it from the side-lines. I had made it further than anticipated, both in terms of my recovery and my personal objectives, but this realisation hit hard. How much recovery was feasible? An open question and a very challenging situation.

The Documentary

As requested by Prof. Dr. Hubert Vermeersch, the surgeon in charge of the facial surgery, I consented to the operation being filmed.

> The main objective of the documentary is to get the word out about the 'Facial Centre', a multidisciplinary unit newly founded at Ghent Hospital for complex facial surgery.
>
> At this department, various surgeons (plastic surgeons, head surgeons and neck surgeons) join forces to take facial surgery to the next level. This is what medical progress is about. Many people can benefit from this, from road traffic victims to people with injuries or facial defects caused by war, violence etc. Moreover, the footage will serve as a teaching resource for surgeons in training.

The hospital had collaborated before with director Bart Beckers from 'Screensavers'.[1] I met with Bart and quickly trusted his vision, which was necessary, because he would also shoot at my home and during a performance of my band, 'Les Cochons Sublimes'. He wanted to involve my personal life in the documentary as well. As the documentary would contribute to medical progress and the hard work of the surgeons, I was quick to agree. However, it did put additional strain on my trajectory and I had to make an additional effort – not an easy feat for someone with my condition.

The Cascade of Necessary Medical Follow-Up

I had to accept that life as I had known it was largely over. The rest of my life, especially the first years, would most likely require a close assessment of my medical condition. The appointments kept coming in, my schedule was fully booked for the next two years and any other events had to be planned in function of all this medical attention.

Many experts had to permanently follow up on my situation. I had to pay regular visits to the ear specialist to have the hearing protection for my right ear (the only one still functioning) checked and the evolution of my damaged balancing organ assessed. A 'cross system' to divert all incoming sound to my right ear was the only viable option, since my left ear was simply too damaged to be accommodated by a classical hearing aid. My eyes had recovered quite a lot, but I couldn't close my left one anymore, so I paid regular visits to the ophthalmologist as well. Additionally, there were the routine appointments with my neurologist, who visually mapped the evolution of my brain, would monitor the shunt for the rest of my life and regularly re-evaluated the dosage of my epilepsy medication. The neurosurgeon, in turn, would evaluate the blood flow in my skull on a regular basis and, in case of further tissue necrosis, intervene surgically. The many scars on my body and skin required extra attention, as did my reconstructed urethra…

'Le Grand tour de l'UZ Gent doit se répéter pour une durée indéterminée', the grand tour of Ghent Hospital has to go on indefinitely… Still, I was determined to accept this turn of events: long live medical science and the therapeutic support carefully tailored to my situation.

Note

1 A Belgian production company.

Reference

Verplaetse, Jan (2008) *Het morele instinct*. Amsterdam: Nieuwezijds.

Chapter 4

Mental Recovery

Unstable Consciousness, Energy Deficit and Radical Reset

Over the course of a couple of months, my mental state had evolved from completely comatose to semi-comatose and, ultimately, mostly conscious. This transition ushered in an era of unthinkable challenges in quick succession, a transformation of my trusted flat open country into a rugged, mountainous terrain. My talent for optimism was now on the line in the face of what could well be years of struggle. The word 'IMPAIRMENT' made its capital entry into my personal vocabulary. My career as a teacher in special-needs education had already familiarised me with the concept of 'IMPAIRMENT' and had given me the opportunity to teach at schools for children with mild (Reynaertschool, Ghent) or serious (Blijdorp, Buggenhout) mental and physical disabilities. Still, these experiences had not prepared me for the impact of such a personal confrontation.

It became clear early on in recovery that keeping my mental balance would cost a lot of energy, which was already in short supply and continuously in overdemand. One of the hallmarks of ABI, as it turned out, was a persisting feeling of fatigue in combination with a diminished load capacity, or, in terms of energy: more consumption, less supply. This was a very real problem for my mental housekeeping. It kept me from performing daily activities that are considered easy and self-evident under normal circumstances, such as cleaning the table, getting dressed, … Any attempt to vacuum-clean when I came home had to be paid for with a long rest of many hours and just doing groceries brought about an uncontrollable stream of negative stimuli that was hard to process. I felt like a novice housekeeper. It took a lot of time and effort to restore balance in this situation.

As soon as my consciousness allowed me to, I started to notice a daily reset of my mental condition. If my life was a game of Monopoly,

DOI: 10.4324/9781003205142-5

then I always drew a 'Go back to the start' card, only in my case without collecting £200. Recent achievements were often undone as quickly as they came, progress was a matter of going back to square one and the only dynamic that was truly guaranteed was that there would always be a next challenge just around the corner.

All assumptions about life, carefully collected throughout decades, were instantly swept into the trash can. They no longer were relevant or applicable. I found myself in a different reality now, one with its own specific nature and unknown laws. I had only just managed to find peace and quiet as a 40-year-old man. The ramblings and haphazard soul-searching of my youth had made way for determination and acceptance of myself – even of my appearance, despite my increasing age. Now, everything this stage of my life stood for was wiped away. I denied all involvement in 'worldly affairs' for a long time. All I could do was watch from the side – a hermit very much against my will, bereft of all I considered achievements of my willpower.

In times of relapse (numerous as they were), the days were often off to a bad start, for instance after the urethroplastic and facial surgery, or the epileptic attack. The desire for a shift in my emotional perspective to get through the day was stronger then than during any other stage of my recovery. The mental struggle for daily functionality was fierce and intense, as was the resistance against emotional deterioration. It took an enormous effort to keep reacting positively and resiliently to the challenges of the day. I was also quite strict with myself and rarely happy with concrete realisations, for instance in my role as a father. For many months after I came home from the rehab centre, I hardly interacted with my family. The available energy was just enough to 'be' there physically, but socially I resided on my own private island, unresponsively. For my wife and kids, this was a challenging and uncertain situation. Dad was back, but not quite. So I shifted my focus inward to be able to go about my day as well as possible.

On a weekly basis, almost from day to day, both during and after moments of relapse, I was confronted with one depressed emotion or another. They came in different forms and shapes but were always physically noticeable and seemed to be the direct result of either the brain injury or of the changing circumstances in which I found myself. Their exact cause wasn't always clear to me and trying to look into it (as I also did in the case of my willpower and optimism) became a daily occupation. Apart from these philosophical ruminations, I was quite happy with my ability to react so eagerly to the situation. I had the feeling it was something that just happened to me, but I was aware of its potential and wanted to make the most of it. Still, although it allowed me to achieve ambitious goals in my recovery, I often had to surrender newly conquered terrain in part or in full. This roulette of emotions was complicated by the fact that every stage of the recovery came with its own priorities and difficulties. For example:

- There was a stage where I had to regain my daily self-reliance so I could eat solid food and wash without assistance again.
- There were weeks I particularly worried about the condition of my eyes: would I go blind or could I avoid it?
- The replacement of my bone flap required all my focus and energy for weeks.
- It took me weeks to finally get rid of the wheelchair for good, only to find that my muscle mass had eroded by the long period of inactivity.
- At a certain point I had lost more than 20 kg because I couldn't eat. I was at risk of getting malnourished, of losing all chances of recovery, and even of dying. That's when they decided to supplement through tube-feeding during the nights. For weeks, as long as the tube was in place, there simply was no room for working on any of my other objectives.

My short-term memory was yet another part of me affected by the injury. So much energy went into many frustrating searches for lost keys, pens, handkerchiefs, eye drops or sunglasses. Even keeping my grocery bag or workspace organised proved to be a messy and complicated affair. At times, when things got busy, I often lost oversight of the course of the day and had to call on my wife and others to constantly restructure time and space.

For a while it seemed I would no longer be able to drive a car. When it turned out this might still be possible after all, I went all out. I completed an extensive driving test to prove my brain injury didn't prevent me from driving safely and responsibly. After the epileptic attack, my license was again revoked until I could prove I did not suffer any attacks for six months through written attestation of my doctor. It's safe to say a lot of effort went into reclaiming this part of my independence. However, being a passenger in a car came with its own set of difficulties. No more radio, because it led to overstimulation and a heavy head, in part because of the hearing impairment, but mostly due to my dysfunctional stimulus processing. The sound of the engine in combination with the ever-changing traffic situation and the fact it wasn't me who was driving kept me constantly on edge. The noise of the radio was more than I could handle.

The further I got in recovery, the more I sighed, literally. It took a lot explaining to people that I wasn't angry or irritated: it was simply the easiest and fastest way for my body to relax, especially in moments of time pressure or stimulus overload. Often, I didn't feel bad, I just had to let off steam to keep my focus and to use my endurance to the fullest, a deep sigh to mentally prepare for long, continuous exertion – be it vacuuming, writing, cleaning a table or driving. The sighing only grew stronger as more objectives were completed.

Preserving My Personality

During the first year after the accident, I developed ways to be resilient in the face of changing circumstances. The need for resilience only grew over the course of my volatile recovery.

There were especially four things that systematically fuelled that resilience: my warm and loving family, the fact I was back at playing music, working towards becoming a long-distance runner and the support of my parents and friends.

Besides these external motivators, there also was an intrinsic reason why I could maintain a decent level of optimism from the very start: I was under the impression that I had managed to preserve most of my personality – which is no small blessing for someone with a brain injury as severe as mine. The worst example I had witnessed with my own eyes at the rehab centre was a mother who didn't recognise her own child anymore. The fact that I had narrowly escaped a similar fate made me feel relieved. I made peace with this feeling – because of, but also in spite of, the fact that others weren't so lucky. I didn't take any pleasure in the misery of those less fortunate than I and I would sooner watch a soap opera than enjoy the drama of those suffering a fate similar to mine.

I focussed as hard as I could on my own situation and tried to experience just how much of me was left. The brain damage was undeniable and was initially especially discernible in the shape of my failing short-term memory and my weak concentration. I tried to assess which aspects were due to the brain damage and which ones were attributable to the changing circumstances.

Fortunately, those around me soon confirmed with conviction that I was still very much the same person with the same character and temperament. The first to do so were my wife and kids. Because they were so convinced of the fact, I was too. Who else could give me this much certainty? We were lucky: our family got its husband and father back, which immediately led to deep feelings of gratitude. It was no superficial 'hip-hip-hooray' moment: it was a profound feeling of relief at the realisation that I was still here.

Moreover, I wasn't alienated from acquaintances and the history we had in common. I managed to get my bearings relatively quickly when entering a social circle. I recognised neighbours, colleagues and their position at work. I could recall multiple informal contacts and the small talk we had exchanged in the past.

However, this time as well I was determined to be realistic and to face the truth: besides these reassuring observations, some things about me had truly changed. Recalling names was often challenging, even of those I had seen on a daily basis for a certain period. This led to awkward moments and feelings of uncertainty. Also finding my way through the house turned out to be challenging and I often wound up in the kitchen when looking for the hallway or stairs and vice versa. Along with my forgetfulness of the songs of my band, 'Les Cochons Sublimes', these were the most remarkable examples of my memory loss. Luckily, things got better with time and kept improving for a long while.

What's more, my mental mechanics were more inclined to create structure and my focus became more specific. This became apparent in my lesson preparations as a teacher and my style as a bass player. I had also developed a compulsive urge to achieve predefined goals and a greater need for predictability. Not much was left of my carelessness with which I did things before the accident. Still, I stubbornly tried to get the most out of these sudden changes in my identity.

It became clear that a big part of my essence had been preserved. The fundamental traits of my personality had not been rooted out by the damage of the accident. Still, I had to face the truth: I was left with a serious brain injury and it would surely have a great, discernible impact on the course of my life and the development of my identity. Just how much only time could tell.

The realisation that neurological processes lie at the heart of one's identity fills me with persistent doubt. My neurological system has changed a lot: does this mean I am someone else now? I see all life as matter, so too conscious life, but in the case of my own consciousness this demonstrable observation is quite the shock. The brain lesion of my right temporal lobe changes the matter related to thought. If thinking is only a matter of matter, then the accident must have an enormous influence on my existence. To talk about myself in terms of brain activity is counterintuitive. Am I nothing more than mere brain activity? No, I am not. It takes a lot of effort to emotionally accept this logical paradigm. Its conclusions have great consequences for my perception of man in general, but especially for my self-image and my own journey.

I have to control my fear of losing control of myself and to get as realistic and constructive an understanding of my situation as possible. Writing (and reading) helps. I try to assess to the best of my abilities the similarities and differences in personality before and after the accident.

Existential Loneliness

Because of the severity and inevitability of the situation, various (often conflicting) observations took centre stage.

First and foremost, there was the daily realisation that I was surrounded by the right people, those who went the extra mile to be there for me. Despite that proximity, the unavoidable distance was continuously palpable. No matter how things would turn out, life would go on for other people, regardless of whether I would be conscious, alive or neither. This realisation truly confronted me with a feeling of isolation. I often decided not to ruminate on it for too long and to just accept it. Sometimes all this felt like a great mental show of force.

This feeling really took hold when I returned to my 'second home'. In the teachers' lounge, I noticed that I had drifted away from life's epicentre. All work-related events and dynamics took place independent of my recovery and existence. I had trouble following some of the conversations, a weird sensation for someone who had been at the heart of operations for years. I wanted to collaborate and be part of the organisation again. In spite of the warm welcome from my colleagues, at times, I couldn't help but feel alone during breaks. It would take time before I'd be a fully-fledged employee again. I could hardly wait.

Isolation can also have practical causes, as is the case for me. My feelings of loneliness are amplified by the permanent hearing impairment. In big groups with chaotic communication, it takes a lot of effort and energy to keep up. I have to position myself strategically to discern conversations and to join them. People on my left, for instance, are often unintelligible. To make matters worse, my diminished load capacity has a hard time processing multiple stimuli at the same time. An unfortunate, permanent outcome of my ordeal, and a big contrast to what was before: I used to thrive in big audiences and loved to drift from one conversation or group to another. This has become well-nigh impossible.

As if things weren't already hard enough, reality made it painfully clear to me once again: I had to make it by myself without getting depressed – that would do no good, on the contrary, it would make things even more difficult for me and those around me. Feelings of depression increase the distance between myself and others and would be very counterproductive in a situation of life and death. In this, my talent for mental optimism found one of its toughest challenges. There was hard work to be done. It was a matter of life and death.

This realisation strengthened my belief that to approach this matter with positive willpower was the only workable option, if only for selfish reasons: I would be able to count on maximum support if I persevered wholeheartedly, because it would make it easier for others to keep on investing their time in me.

Time and Desire

Confronted with an unsolicited retardation of my life, I was forced to find new meaningful ways of living my life. There wasn't much left of what once was. I was overwhelmed by a sudden sea of emptiness amidst all the time I had to spare, time that irrevocably went by while I passively watched it slip away. Although this void was not my own fault, accepting it was nonetheless hard and I felt bad giving in to it. An important part of my recovery therefore was to find new content and to reactivate myself to the extent this was still possible. I started writing, reading, running, working and caring for the kids as far as possible. Oftentimes, the results were minimal, but I carried on regardless, because doing nothing would truly mean and feel like defeat.

In the first months after the accident, I was forced to do nothing for hours on end. My body could only rest, either tied to the bed or not. At a later stage, my hunger for action still remained unsatisfied because of the energy deficit and the diminished load capacity. To get past that and seek solutions was a long-term endeavour. I hadn't chosen to rest, but I was in need of it anyway, given that all available energy went to my body fighting back against unfavourable odds. The first year, there was no room for anything else. The situation changed continuously throughout recovery, but my diminished load capacity was constant. I lived in another reality.

At many moments, time seemed to stretch out into the vast, immeasurable void. It simply would not pass. I lay there waiting, months and months of waiting, waiting for caretakers, for therapy, for visitors, for surgery, for blended food, for doctor's appointments, for the night to be over, for signs of recovery …

For the most part, I was on my own, confronted with great loneliness and pointlessness. I often had to fight not to give up. Luckily, I still had my family and friends. I also developed the growing conviction that a meaningful life goes hand in hand with forms of pure pointlessness. The sheer triviality of the accident amply demonstrated this. I learned how to use that realisation as a liberating strength: all value is to be found in isolated moments, in the here and now, face to face with people.

My run-in with existential emptiness drove my mind to a multitude of unexpected thoughts and desires. The freed-up space was continuously filled with restless musings. My brain used the situation to produce new connections, ideas and imaginations, embracing its 'second life', as it were, and making the most of the compulsory rest of my body. It drew on less-used aspects of my personality to start again.

In this context, I came across an interesting quote by Blaise Pascal[1] that was mentioned by Ignaas Devisch[2] in an interview on the human tendency towards desire and restlessness.

> In his Pensées, Pascal elaborately describes the tension between ennui and entertainment, boredom and confusion. In my view, he captures the essence in one of his most famous quotes: man is not able to quietly sit in an empty chamber. It is not as much the circumstances that agitate us, according to Pascal, but something in our nature that forces us to act. We cannot stop desire by isolating ourselves from stimuli and social contacts, because that would render our life perspectiveless and meaningless. Hence, he does not believe we can get to a point of total detachment. Man will always pursue and desire. At the same time, he isn't lucid enough to see that this lands him in a conflict where he is torn between the urge to act and the feeling of lacking time to realise his ambitions.
>
> (Ignaas Devisch in Knack, March 24, 2016)

I knew the feeling of being urged to act all too well. It meant that I sometimes felt insatiable, stressed and under immense time pressure – something I could hardly handle anymore. However, the advantage that more than outdid the drawbacks was that I became highly motivated. I had to do things here and now, with conviction and perseverance. The fact I was given a second life was absolutely exceptional, and this realisation made my decisiveness soar to new heights.

My motivation was rooted in the realisation that all things valuable come from contemporary reality. Moreover, my eagerness seemed to be continuously fuelled by instinctive motivators inherent to my body. I had to use it wisely, despite the complicated circumstances, and for that, I had to look into the nature and origin of my desires. I craved detachment from life outside myself and circumstances free from stimuli on a thorough search for a workable balance between my extroversion and my radically new reality. I had to find a way to engage in constructive restlessness and to temper its exhausting counterpart (special thanks in this regard to 'Rusteloosheid' ('Restlessness') by Ignaas Devisch (Devisch, 2016) – for the useful inspiration complementary to my own the experience).

I learned to understand the world outside the dominant concept of time:

> Life is not a linear journey to one goal or another that ultimately determines its value. There is no 'life plan', neither for society nor for the individual, we are not necessarily bound for some sort of 'wholesome afterlife', a 'pure nation', 'continuous economic growth' or even impressive careers and material wealth'. To think so would be an illusion.

I was thrown upon a different experience of time, one in which progress came with relapse, where past and future were understood as mere imaginations in the ever-unfolding present. Time was no longer a coherent structure with a start and a finishing line, nor something with limited availability in which realisations are scarce by definition. My impairments gave me another perspective on the course of reality. The 'now' became bigger and constituted my main angle of approach to look at the past and future. My thoughts were less directed to the realisation of a scheme for the future and I thoroughly perceived the restless nature of permanent change. Time felt untameable and unpredictable and I had to accept that my recovery would be long and its outcome uncertain. Mentally, it was a huge challenge to live with manifest and acute impairments.

I felt a growing resistance against extreme desires. Resistance against forced-upon needs such as wealth or status had been part of my temperament before, but now it flared up amidst these changing circumstances. I felt well-nigh immune to excess and kept a rein on my nonetheless insatiable drive.

Another illustration of how reaching mental balance remained a big challenge: I felt the urge to take over absolute control from my desires. Life became an exercise in letting go, letting go of my past self, of life as I had known it, of old priorities and former plans. A good friend once told me that letting go is one of the most important but also one of the most difficult skills in life. Under these extreme circumstances, this became all the more true. I was forced with immediate effect to reform my identity. My cognitive workings had changed as well and made room for different neural networks that brought new balance to my consciousness. The existing structure mostly remained intact, but was now supplemented and corrected by an unexpected, extreme event. The meaning of a successful and valuable life had evolved dramatically. Despite this thorough change, fortunately, I could still recognise myself in an authentic way.

Dealing with Fate and Bad Luck

Without warning, I was forced to deal with a multitude of unfortunate events. I could have gotten stuck and wallowed in feelings of injustice, injustice as the new cornerstone of my developing personality, victimhood as the new motor of my existence: 'look at me, I'm broken ...' Fortunately, I had no desire to be guided by any of these things and actively resisted them, even though something had happened that had made me a victim and in which I had no part.

Which attitude did I have to undergo the unavoidable with? Did I have any choice at all? Could I take any credit whatsoever for my talent for mental optimism or was this just a genetically, neurologically and hormonally predetermined situation, an innate temperament or trait that might just as well have been different?

That last question was always on my mind. I became convinced that I needed to consciously appropriate a way to deal with the situation. I didn't have a say in the fact that I had to deal with the situation in the first place, but at the very least I would reserve the right to decide my reaction for myself. This became a constant object of deliberation. Did I have any influence over my attitude? Maybe there were some options to determine the way in which I was driven by the inevitable. It seemed hard, but not impossible, as did governance over my own interpretation of the facts.

I spent more and more time thinking about this problem, looking for ways to go about it. It felt like a general human experience. By talking about my situation, I noticed how often people wind up in demanding scenarios. More often than I would have guessed, life seemed to be a confrontational experience. More likely than not, ill fortune will strike in most people's lives sooner or later. On the one hand, I knew that my anecdotal perspective did not justify a generalised conclusion, it's just that this kind of topic was often brought up in my presence because of my own situation. On the other hand, it is a demonstrable fact that life is finite and fragile for all. Indeed, the society of which I was a part still had the privilege of being prosperous and largely resilient against the harshness of reality. I felt like I couldn't complain, despite the difficult circumstances. Refining my way of dealing with the extreme hardships and giving it (if possible) universal utility gradually became a valuable objective to me.

I wanted to transform the insights I had gained through experience into a generally applicable concept for overcoming hurdles in life – an ambitious plan prone to failure, but nonetheless a necessity in my eyes. There was no other choice, it was a matter of survival in a meaningful way. I had set out on a journey with no way back, I had to follow through.

- The question then became: how can I react? There seemed to be a couple of options:
- To ignore the accident. Maybe it would bring about some moments of rest, even if it wouldn't work in the long run.
- To rebel, to vent the frustration, even if I couldn't change the situation.
- To acquiesce, to stop the resistance as a deliberate choice, not from necessity.
- To accept the situation, to simply undergo it, to save my strength.
- To make fun of it all, to create distance from the accident by rising above it, to mitigate the suffering or to reject my victimhood.
- To acknowledge the bad fortune, but to conceive the accident as something positive, for whatever reason.
- To use the bad fortune to my advantage, to make the most of it, to transform it (Schmid, 2005).

Intuitively, I felt most inclined to 'acknowledge and use' the accident and I began to look for ways to do so. How could I become a better teacher, a more thoughtful father, a more valuable friend, a more loving husband, a more interesting writer, …?

I was looking for an opportunistic and optimistic approach and a reversal of this ominous situation. This was my way of dealing with the inevitable, in addition to making fun of the situation – humour as a wrecking ball often worked wonders. What follows in the remainder of this chapter is a description of the strategies and attitudes I resorted to to achieve this reversal.

Language against the Impairment and 'Tested Expressions'

Early in recovery, language started to play an important role. I still loved to speak French as much after as I did before the brain injury.

There was a time during the first weeks after the accident when I communicated exclusively in French – fairly correct French for that matter, or so I was told. Semi-comatose and acutely polyglottic! Also, my kids also immediately noticed their father's affectionate words and expressions. I still called them by their pet names, such as 'oozy-boozy' or 'snotty-wotty'.

I had the motivation and ambition to limit my impairments to a bare minimum, which was a challenging assignment, not least because the physical changes caused by the accident were clearly visible. My face had been thoroughly changed by the partial paralysis of my left side. My left eye was also clearly bigger than my right one because I could no longer move the lid of the former and because the socket of the latter was shattered. This caused my right eye to sink deeper into my face. My mouth was oblique, its left corner immobile and sagging down. At my right temple, there was a 'crater' due to the removal of my bone flap.

Physically, my appearance had changed a lot, so much that I could see doubt in the eyes of strangers. People were visibly wondering whether I was mentally okay and many were hesitant to start a conversation. Even children would gawk at me for a long time.

My first instinct was to react by consciously refining my language – a lot. My vocabulary and syntax served to show that underneath this banged-up skull, there still was an intact neurological landscape and that this battered body was still inhabited by the same resident as the one prior to the accident. It was also a way of compensating for non-verbal cues. The paralysis of my face stopped me from using facial expressions. Even my children had a hard time reading my stern and rigid look. I had to hone my language skills tremendously in order to provide an explanation to go with my non-verbal expression.

As soon as my vision and mental conditions permitted, I started working on lesson preparations to start working as a teacher again. It was far from clear whether I'd ever be able to teach again in the first place, but being caught up in philosophical topics boosted my morale nonetheless. That's where my strong focus on language came in handy. It was a confirmation that cognitively, I was still intact and met the basic requirements to get back to work one day.

I also developed a set of 'tested expressions' I could resort to if I wanted to clarify a complicated situation for myself and others. These were phrases that took shape in the months I used them and through which I set the pace for my reactions and behaviour and gave them the right weight. To develop a workable mindset, I was as much in need of stable forms of expression as I required effective and well-advised action. A large number of these expressions contributed to the development of my mental resilience. For instance:

- I tried not to make any problems if there were none and, if there already were problems, not to make them any bigger than strictly necessary.
- Push the boundaries without crossing them in order to avoid or reduce relapse.
- First distance, then speed (in the context of complicated objectives, such as running a marathon or my long recovery). Slowly and steadily stepping up the pace is the best guarantee for a smooth journey without fallbacks.
- Rehabilitation puts me close to / on the same level as professional sports.
- The way we react to things that happen to us is partly up to us. Within the confinements of our character and the circumstances, there is a small but significant space in which we can operate to give direction to our responses. This is the true reach of human cognition and emotion, rooted in natural selection.
- To stress and to reproach drains a lot of energy from my broken body. I try to avoid it whenever I can for the sake of my recovery and managing my load capacity. My immediate surroundings are better off with a tranquil version of myself.

Favourable Circumstances and Unexpected Advantages

In order to be able to believe in a worthy recovery and a meaningful existence, I often focussed on positive evolutions and remaining possibilities. I was constantly on the look-out for the favourable side of things, though I often had to explain to myself, my wife and those around me what this favourable side exactly was. People thought these circumstances were far from favourable, and indeed, in a sense they were. Still, I often felt the urge to jokingly clarify this claim with the words of the 'famous philosopher' Johan Cruyff: 'every cloud 'as its silver lining'[3]. So given the circumstances, I gladly pointed out the following:

- My family proved to be rock-solid, even in the worst of times.
- My mental condition made getting back to work a distinct possibility. Since my job gave meaning to my life and I could count on a lot of appreciation from pupils and colleagues, this was a great prospect indeed.

- I could play music again with my band. Clearly, processing multiple stimuli was still possible under the right circumstances!
- My parents and closest friends did everything within their power to get me through this. I was in exceptionally good company.
- I still recognised myself and had managed to preserve most of my personality.
- In a relatively short span of time, I had managed to get rid of the wheelchair, staggering persistently to a more stable future.
- Physically, a meaningful recovery was still possible. The road seemed rocky and long, but on it led regardless, towards significant improvement.
- The brain training improved thanks to my musical and linguistic activities.

With time, moreover, came unexpected perspectives on the circumstances and I soon began to realise that not only were there mitigating circumstances in my ordeal, there were also even advantages. The effect was not unlike the known phenomenon of unforeseen, perverted results of far-reaching decisions.

Powerful politicians know this phenomenon all too well from political decision-making. Good intentions and prestigious realisations oftentimes lead to counterproductive and unwanted side-effects. A couple of examples:

- When medical insurance covers hospital fees but not the prevention costs, this might encourage people to live an unhealthier life. Prevention costs money, so the implicit reasoning goes, but being in hospital doesn't.
- Tax increases can harm the economy, because taxpayers will be closer to their spending limit or migrate to other countries, resulting in lower tax revenues at a later stage.
- If a government bans drugs out of health or ethical concerns, this stimulates an illegal circuit that makes the drugs harder to control and therefore all the more dangerous.

In my situation, I was confronted with the inverse of this phenomenon: even though no one would voluntarily choose it for that reason, the dramatic situation seemed to come with certain unexpected advantages. Albeit counterintuitive and coincidental, these consequences, unlike their negative counterparts, were not completely undesirable. What follows are some examples of this observation.

First, my wife and I became more aware of our love for each other. We gave more attention to one another at a time when our intimate connection needed a thorough revaluation. At the same time, I became more easy-going and less demanding in friendships.

I enjoyed the little things more than ever – filling a bird feeder in our garden, for example. As long as the feeder was full, I got better. It became the symbolic measuring device of my own recovery. Also, I had been without my driving licence for months, until the day I got it back from a driving instructor and was allowed to drive again. I was over the moon. As a final example: the collateral damage of the accident included a damaged urethra, to a point where surgery was necessary to prevent a total blockage of my urinary tract. I had to wait for this surgery for two months – an enormous weight pressing down on my shoulders, as if the brain injury in itself wasn't already enough. It was one of the moments I learned what injustice feels like. I never would have guessed I'd be as happy as a clam by just standing upright and relieving myself at a urinal after a successful operation. I remember it as if it were only yesterday and urinating at a urinal has remained a source of joy ever since.

A year after the accident, I had recovered enough to attend a two-day philosophical seminar in Leuven and in the De Krook library in Ghent. In Leuven, there was a discussion on the place of philosophy and philosophising in secondary education, whereas the topic at Ghent was the legacy of May '68:[4] what was left of the '60s idealism of fighting authority with imagination? Can philosophers change the world? Before the accident, I would have never dared to speak in the presence of such 'big thinkers' in the audience. One of the potential consequences of an ABI, however, is a diminished sense of restraint. Usually, this is negative and comes in the shape of coarse language or sexually inappropriate behaviour, but in this case, it led to a contribution to a philosophical debate – definitely one of the positive ways the impairment can manifest itself. I took the stage both in Leuven and Ghent to defend the idea of philosophy as an attitude.

My personal opinion: philosophical conversations provide pupils in secondary education with the opportunity to learn to disagree in a safe environment – an essential skill in times of superdiversity. 'Our society is evolving into a forum of ever-growing dissent', according to one of the philosophers at the seminar in Ghent. It immediately made me aware of the didactic role of philosophy. Philosophical thought and speech can serve as a reference point in dealing with diversity: if you hear a controversial opinion, don't just stop listening, but team up with that person in a temporary 'research community' in which you explore the value of the arguments together.

I didn't need alcohol anymore to loosen up in socially overwhelming circumstances: my brain injury took care of that and became a 'socialising agent'. My continuous processing and elaborating of ideas was also a consequence of the decreased sense of restraint.

At a certain point in my recovery, I became a role model, whether I liked it or not. Apparently, the optimistic way in which I dealt with my fate made an impression on those who witnessed it. Also, out of nowhere, I became an expert in brain-related injury – a true asset in my line of work.

I seemed to have 'time to spare', which I used to find new social networks and to restore the old ones, as well as to fully invest in me, my family and my recovery. Those sharing my fate at K7 in Ghent Hospital in particular were valuable additions to my social network. For months, we went through a similar demanding trajectory and many of us kept in touch afterwards. Our connection developed amidst difficult but deeply human circumstances. Their resilience and willpower were impressive proof of human perseverance. It took me more than a year to truly connect with others, but when I pulled it off, it turned out to be really valuable. In May 2018, when I performed with my band in a pub called 'Volkshuis' in Ghent, some people from K7 came to watch the show. This was a new experience: finally, I integrated socially again.

At the same time, I tried to renew old connections. I noticed that I had a different way of approaching people I had known before, starting from a new, refreshing perspective on our common background. By virtue of our interaction, I discovered the differences and similarities with my former self and how these evolutions related to one another.

For the first time in my life, I had the feeling that thoughts and words kept coming, without interruption – an inconvenient experience at times, especially when I tried to go to sleep, but also a perk when it came to writing. Also, I hardly ever got bored …

Making the Difference

Without any pretence at achieving lofty, ground-breaking ambitions, it was nonetheless really important for my self-worth to have the opportunity to make a difference. This was already the case before the accident and I had pulled it off at the time in a couple of ways. Now that I had regained consciousness, I found out how exactly. It became clear from what my friends, colleagues and even pupils and their parents told me, from the letters they gave to my wife and later from the visits they paid me at the rehabilitation centre. Thank you all! When my wife first read the letters, I said 'so I did leave a trace after all', one of the few occasions I actually spoke at the time. Still, the nature and potential of the life ahead was highly uncertain.

The visits and writings of those people and their firm conviction which they asserted my value with have been of utmost importance for my recovery. They assured me of the meaningfulness of my struggle. The road ahead was long, but these people gave it direction.

Among them are a couple of enormously talented people with their heart in the right place, by the way …

It was an absolute pick-me-up that kept me from looking at humanity with negative feelings due to the circumstances. On the contrary: my faith in the power and security of social connections even increased.

However trite everything may seem when explained by evolution, the importance of the now and the meaningfulness therein defines the essence and true value of life. My awareness of that fact has only grown since my ABI. It's a search known to all who crave for a balance between rest and motivation in the modern age, and I seem to represent a rather 'extreme' version of this trope.

Moreover, the 'helper's high' I derived from this wonderful feedback motivated me to go beyond just 'making a difference': I also wanted to make *as much* difference as humanly possible. Inspired by the philosophy of Effective Altruism,[5] I decided that the profits of this book should go to one of the most effective charitable causes, as identified through thorough empirical and scientific screening. As mentioned before, the circumstances of my ordeal were all in all favourable and I owe a lot to our social welfare and medical technology. Unfortunately, most sentient life on earth isn't so lucky and cannot rely in the same way on the mercy of science, social security or material prerequisites for lasting happiness. As one of the richest people ever on this planet (as is the vast majority of those living in the West for that matter), I see it as my duty to spend at least some of my time and resources on trying to create the favourable conditions which all are entitled to but many are bereft of due to the Russian roulette of life. Therefore, after careful deliberation, I chose Eight.world, because their unconditional cash transfers to the extremely poor has been proven to be one of the most effective ways to alleviate challenging human circumstances. Moreover, the organisation was founded by people from my hometown – I even went to school with one of them!

And then the icing on the cake: the translator of my manuscript proposed the compensation for his work would go entirely to Animal Charity Evaluators' Recommended Charity Fund – a fund that allocates its capital in a scientifically calculated manner to the charities that are most effective at reducing animal suffering.

'Yes, but, Then Again, I Have a Brain Injury, You Know'

The longer I work on this text, the more I notice I tend to mix the present tense with the preterit. Different themes quickly succeed one another and are often set out simultaneously. And then there's the repetition, which I allow myself to give into from a healthy form of opportunism and with a certain sense of humour – and which I shamelessly dare to reflect upon in said text! I try to resolve the issue by adapting the lay-out and refining the structure as much as possible. To meticulously organise things seems to have become a mandatory attitude in all aspects of my life.

Any potential criticism I conveniently ward off with the following 'cynical' joke: 'yes but, then again, I have a brain injury, you know.' I've been milking this comeback for a while now in order to have the final say. I guess by now I've squeezed every last drop out of it.

The expression became a running gag after recovery. I knew beforehand that this dark sense of humour wouldn't be appreciated by everyone. I imagined that those sharing my faith might have some problems with it. That's why I used the expression sparingly and only in a safe context. I didn't really mean it, of course, but it helped me put things into perspective.

The Counterproductivity of Fear and Useful Rancour: The Transformation of Emotions

The accident and its consequences (such as the epileptic attack more than a year later) forced me to continuously worry about the functioning of my brain. Going down so uncontrollably and unexpectedly had made a deep impression on me and I wanted to avoid its repetition at all costs, so I radically adapted my behaviour and choices. I immediately stopped drinking, knowing that this could be a trigger for epilepsy, which in itself was sufficient a reason to quit.

The fear of another 'short circuit' was deeply ingrained and became the symbolic focal point of all my anxieties about the ABI and related injuries. Of course, to act out of fear seemed to me a bad idea that would only amplify the impairments of my life. Fortunately, I couldn't call it a disorder yet, but fear was one of the emotions I had to learn to control as far as possible and that I started to consider as a useful ally, out of necessity. Fear has strengthened my talent for moderation and I have given the feeling its rightful place through rational reflection.

As such, I fought all forms of excessive fear, for instance by taking to the road by bike fairly early on. At the rehab centre, I learned to ride a bike again, first on a tricycle, then on a bicycle. Ghent Hospital turned out to be equipped with a big network of underground corridors, which became the terrain of my practice sessions. I suppressed feelings of fear and eventually managed to get back on the road again. Reactions of others that were driven by fear I accepted understandingly but refuted firmly with the following 'tested expression': 'If you allow life to be governed by fear, then in a way, you cease to exist.' This was quite a radical view of the facts, but nonetheless completely necessary given the numerous factors that constrained me. To me, this was a form of nonviolent resistance: the only thing I had some control over were my own behaviour and views. I followed through on this resistance by forcing myself to act, especially when experiencing oppressive feelings.

The hardest part was to keep my fear of additional setbacks in check. I didn't feel like I had enough energy or resilience left for that, so the possibility of newly emerging difficulties made me very anxious. I often wondered whether I had to accept that the best part of my life was over and that now was the era of sorrow and ill fortune. That fear persisted and kept surfacing even at later stages of my recovery. However, it was pointless to allow my acts and thoughts to be guided by this. First, the fear hadn't been realised, so this was something to hold on to. Second, I couldn't control the outcomes of my situation, so worrying about it was an unaffordable waste of energy already in short supply.

I had to transform the emotional side of my reaction to drastic events into a form of rational consideration. It was of the utmost importance to get back to a good life. I tried to direct my emotions towards my recovery and spent much energy on trying to look at reality fearlessly and with hope. I was in a most uncertain situation, but kept believing in the possibility of a happy ending, with which I tried to align my most dominant and most frequent thoughts – fear, anger, rancour, feelings of injustice, powerlessness, hope, attachment, love, friendship, unrest, sadness, guilt, doubt, ...

In the direst of moments, I leveraged my principal concern: the future of my daughters. To my mind, a resilient and emotionally stable father would provide the best framework for a steady development of their young lives.

> Emotions play an important role in interpreting facts and events. There is a cognitive side to them (special thanks to Martha Nussbaum[6] for revealing the fact to me) that allows us to steer and use them to our advantage and to that of those around us. Oftentimes, this is difficult, but nonetheless possible. Emotion and rationality are not dualistic opposites: they are complementary expressions of the workings of our brain.
>
> During my recovery, I read in 'The Ancestor's Tale' by Richard Dawkins and Yan Wong (Dawkins and Wong, 2017) that our last common ancestor with another species (chimpanzees or bonobos) lived approximately six million years ago. Just to be clear: we do not descend from bonobos, but from an evolutionary perspective, we share a rather recent common ancestor. During the millions of years that followed, our brains have gradually gone their separate ways, without premeditation and with the help of certain random changes. This has led to our unique way of dealing with rationality and emotions and to the complex abilities of our brain.

I often felt strengthened by a special and sudden feeling of useful rancour. It proved to be key in the fight for preservation. I managed to feel a controlled form of rage against the circumstances, without wasting energy on counterproductive ways of venting. On the contrary: it was a source of energy. I called it 'a specialist's way of fighting back'. I made sure not to take my frustration and anger out on others, but to only use it for fighting the physical and mental impairments instead.

Even the drunk driver who nearly killed me escaped my wrath. I refused to waste energy on it and tried to deal with the circumstances as rationally as possible: wasting energy is not rational. I learned that holding a grudge only thwarted my own recovery. Even though the driver was responsible for a wrong decision with disastrous outcomes, a first-instinct emotional reaction to the fact had fewer positive than negative contributions to make to the situation, so I didn't spend a second more on pondering her responsibility. My anger had different priorities now. Transforming rancour into something useful would be very challenging, but I had the feeling I would make it. I often reasserted this impression with the following 'tested expression': 'It is both reasonable and productive to go through life with as few grudges as possible.'

My hard confrontation with reality forced me to accept the anger and fear on my path. This changed my conception of reality and put my talent for optimism in a different position. My hopeful attitude became more pragmatic and sophisticated. It was no vain or utopian construct, but a viable and useful concept, a lifeline in complicated circumstances. Anger, fear and feelings of injustice often surfaced, so I tried to come up with useful interpretations of what was happening to me. Anger made me fight harder, injustice honed my rationality. I accepted the existence of meaningless injustice but also celebrated my coincidentally large resilience by hitting back non-stop, hour after hour, day by day, only relenting to take necessary and stimuli-poor breaks that would increase my overall output. I was obsessed with finding meaningful ways to spend my time. Lost days meant loss of life. Boundaries existed to impose my well-thought-out will upon, empty moments to be overcome by emotional and rational balance, ambition out of necessity.

Philosophy as a Rehab Coach

The history of philosophy is a constant expression of how to deal with confrontational reality, a gigantic stream of almost personal experiences with losses and gains, captured in words. My accident freed up a lot of time to work my way through some of them and to find useful tools therein.

At a certain point, I found much solace in the Stoic interpretation of happiness: 'There is only one way to happiness and that is to cease worrying about things which are beyond the power of our will' (Epictetus).[7]

> A very articulate maxim, but nonetheless hard to put into practice, as I came to experience throughout my ordeal. It requires a specific sort of talent and an extensive set of the right character traits, which makes the choice not as free as it seems to be at first sight.

Still, it was Stoicism and the inspiring movement of Modern Stoicism[8] that fuelled my mental resilience reflex, allowing me to separate event from belief and consequent emotion, and claim the right to interpret reality the way I deemed valuable. In fact, all initiative of choices made and tactics adopted as mentioned in this book can be traced back to this principle. Its importance cannot be overstated. I have experienced its usefulness and seamless transition from theory to practice in an organic and spontaneous way.

In addition, I was inspired by the work of evidence-based believers in progress, in particular by that of Maarten Boudry[9] from Ghent. One of his most important books, 'Illusies voor gevorderden' ('An Advanced Guide to Illusions') (Boudry, 2015) has contributed a lot to my recovery, as becomes clear from some of the views in my own manuscript.

My situation proves that a positive attitude founded on reason is valuable in at least two respects: it has a higher yield than surrender to negativity would have, and it stimulates the involvement from those around you. Moreover, according to me, it is also empirically observable that willpower and faith in a positive outcome lead to better results. With a long way ahead of me, this realisation is vital for my recovery. The fact that modern civilisation has achieved unparalleled progress inspires confidence in a happy ending for my personal situation. Never before was there so little violence, equality between men and women has greatly improved in many different countries, poverty is on the decline globally and, on the same note, medical technology has given me a valuable and meaningful life to look forward to.

I needed a rational, moderate and pragmatic form of optimism. I had no use for naive utopias, semi-religious prophecies and idle dreams of what I could still achieve: I wanted a realistic trajectory. I started from what was still possible in practice and adapted my choices and priorities to the reality of the situation. The following tested expression was used to describe it: 'I don't want to be a naive optimist, but a motivated rational optimist.'

For this approach, I found valuable insights in the writings of people such as Jan Verplaetse,[10] Etienne Vermeersch,[11] Maarten Boudry, Johan Braeckman,[12] Ignaas Devisch and Ico Maly.[13] I had taken many classes from Johan Braeckman as a student. He taught me the potential pitfalls that come with our extensive cognitive abilities.

Johan explains the value of critical thinking, raises awareness for logical fallacies and has helped me understand the importance of thinking 'carefully' (in my own words). Many logical mistakes are inherent to human psychology and as such, making them is neither shameful nor unheard of. By keeping this in mind, we can resist this phenomenon more effectively and become more rational. Some examples of not thinking 'carefully' enough are:

- creating intuitive connections where in truth none exist (such as superstition, irrational feelings of guilt, pseudo-science);
- searching persistently for an unconditional confirmation of one's own point of view without any regard for potential counter-arguments (confirmation bias);
- selecting information based on easy accessibility rather than looking deeper for less salient insights, for instance forming one's opinions solely based on personal experience (availability bias);
- …

To me, a clear understanding of human cognition was an added value to a successful recovery that at the same time provided me with an opportunity to teach something interesting to my pupils.

I was fortunate enough to rediscover the power of literature and so, a good deal of my spare time was taken up with reading. As such, I discovered that Maarten Boudry, a rational thinker with a well-substantiated way of making a point, was (to my mind) nonetheless prone to 'youthful enthusiasm'. For example: in his defence of the liberal welfare state, at some point, he uses phrasings that may come across as little nuanced and emotional, beyond sober objectivity. He calls our society 'superior' to other societies, for which he was criticised by many. His goal was to stress the enormous value of the principles of radical Enlightenment, such as universal human rights, equality of the sexes, freedom of speech, the abolition of slavery, … However, by choosing an eye-catching word that has a negative, elitist and emotional connotation, he is at risk of losing persuasiveness. I see parallels with my own run-in with over-enthusiasm back in days of my first marathon, when the unprepared acceleration after 33 km did me in and led to severe muscle fatigue. The experience has taught me that carefully distributing my energy and pragmatically stepping up the pace is of utmost importance to achieve the best possible results. I couldn't allow myself to give in to such a mistake after the accident. The controversy surrounding Maarten's word choice has sired the following tested expression:

> 'Avoid causing problems where there are none. Do not make problems that are already there bigger than they have to be.'

Then again, maybe Maarten doesn't mind that much. After all, he wants to open up the debate starting from his sceptical insights and belief in progress. Maybe he deliberately wants to cause problems where there aren't any to determine the focus of the debate. This might be an exceptionally valuable and effective perspective. In that case, the title might as well have been 'An Advanced Guide to Distribution' instead of 'An Advanced Guide to Illusions' ... The art of distribution could also significantly increase the growth margin of Maarten's ambitions. Of course, no parallel can ever be drawn with 100% accuracy, but there is nonetheless a clear similarity with the realisations of my recovery.

On Maarten's blog, I read that Steven Pinker[14] gave him a similar tip from another angle. It piqued my interest in Steven's own experience with similar situations and I decided to ask him if ever I would see him again. As it so happened, I had already run into him in a coffee bar in Ghent and we had had a long, enjoyable conversation – a beautiful moment during my 'reintegration' in society and a stroke of luck (yes, it exists!) – so to my mind, there would be more opportunities for continuing our exchange in the future.

One could say that these philosophers (along with Karl Popper, Stijn Bruers, Daniel C. Dennett, Ruben Mersch, Richard Dawkins, Martha Nussbaum, Katrien Devolder, Griet Vandermassen, Alain De Botton, Stephen Greenblatt, Peter Singer ...) were also in a way my mental coaches through their writings. They unknowingly teamed up with the neuropsychologist of Ghent Hospital and established strong 'thinking tracks' in my brain that together grew into an effective cognitive system and the useful perspective on life that I so desperately needed. Fortunately, my rational network had not permanently disintegrated and I was highly motivated to restore it to its former glory, to refine it and even to expand it. I had been working hard on cognitive repair (memory, concentration, attention span, focus ...) in neurotherapy and now, a wonderful tool complemented this effort: philosophy in writing and conversation.

Free Will or Not?

I experienced first-hand that belief in free-will agency can be an important and useful conviction. Even though it may be an illusion (as recent neurological research and philosophical arguments indicate), mentally, it played a crucial role in reconstructing my life, a pawn in the arduous fight for my recovery. I wanted to take back control and have a say in where my life was headed to.

Although I had mostly lost faith in having control over my life due to the extreme circumstances weighing down on me, I hadn't collapsed mentally. The fact I was forced to just undergo it had unforeseen side-effects: oddly enough, it made the situation understandable and even acceptable in a way. It reduced my feeling of self-determination to realistic proportions and I was eager to exert control within the confinements of what was possible.

I've become lenient in my rational approach to reality. Even illusions now can have their place and functionality – and thus their value. In that sense, they have become more than mere illusions. As this realisation springs from what I've experienced under difficult circumstances, it is pragmatic rather than idealistic in nature.

On the other hand, it is important to keep the margin of error of my convictions to a bare minimum and to give them the right weight and pace. This way, I turn them into something profitable. That's where this book comes in. In it, I put my views on self-control and my perceptions of my emotions into perspective. I am looking for a helpful approach, after all, and this book contributes to that.

Was self-determination truly possible, not just in general, but especially in this extreme situation?

I went through the inevitable with the zeal of a resistance fighter. Only I lived this life and so, to my mind, only my approach could have any influence over its course. This attitude was amplified by my run-in with existential loneliness. I did count my blessings, however: I was supported by a family that provided me with many opportunities and I belonged to a society with a level of medical progress that is above average.

Even if science demonstrates that free will is a complete illusion, then still my reaction is mine and mine alone, driven by certain hormonal, neurological and genetic factors in response to concrete circumstances. Even if my reaction is not self-determined, then it is still the outcome of an interplay of character, temperament and environment. Intraspecies diversity is an important aspect of evolution and natural selection, and however small or involuntary it may be, it means that my way of dealing with the situation is exclusively mine.

To put it differently: if we were to rule out the existence of free will – scientifically or logically – this wouldn't mean a unique (conscious?) will in the here and now doesn't exist. Perhaps this can be sufficiently meaningful in itself?

It is an undeniable fact that I have demonstrated much willpower and mental resilience, for which I'm grateful: it just so happens to be the case for me and the situation might as well have been completely different. Even if this can be attributed to the causal determinism of my genetic, neurological and hormonal composition, then still I consider it something valuable that I can be proud of. I am well aware this is an intuitive and emotional view, but I dare say that in itself it makes me human in my very own way.

Reading Jan Verplaetse's (2011) 'Zonder Vrije Wil' ('Without Free Will') made me muse even more on free will during my recovery. When my thoughts on the topic became unstoppable, I decided it was time to start talking about it to avoid any potential alienation, misconceptions or feelings of pointlessness. I found the courage to send Jan an email. He replied and we set up a meeting in a coffee bar. I knew that personal contact could be an added value and indeed, our conversation was very pleasant and Jan showed a sincere interest in my story. Later, I went to one of his lectures at the Breinwijzer Festival. Jan truly added substance to the course of my recovery.

I even distilled a previously mentioned 'tested expression' from his work, which I will repeat and elaborate on here, since I use it very often:

> 'I would be as bold as to recommend everyone to live life with as few grudges as possible. Reproach is often to a significant extent unjustified and most of all a waste of energy better spent on achieving positive goals.'

This feels like an essential insight in life, with all its limitations.

The definition and structure of Jan's position is as follows: free will is the ability to freely choose what to do, why and how, in other words: we decide the action, motivation and effort.

People who deny the existence of free will say that all these decisions are determined by an unconscious causal network of the brain (i.e. cause and result). According to them, there are no alternatives such as a free 'soul' or an 'I'. Indeed, neuroscientists haven't found any such thing in their scans. Our 'conscious' decisions are preceded by unconscious processes, as screenings of brain activity clearly demonstrate. 'Free' will is an illusion, because it cannot make any decisions itself – they have already been made unconsciously before. Free will is just the spokesperson, not the CEO.

People who defend free will say that ordinary psychological abilities suffice to determine whether something is your decision (and thus your responsibility) or not. We have rational abilities (open to reason and responsibility) and the ability to control (self-control: the ability to have the will that you want; behaviour regulation: the ability to avoid doing certain actions). Deniers of free will also value these abilities but find them insufficient for responsibility. To feel responsible and to take responsibility is something different from being responsible, which requires control over the source and cause of one's actions and a bigger number of options to choose from. Our self-determination and options are too limited to justify adding 'free' to 'will'. Moreover, we are too prone to manipulation by indoctrination, brainwashing, drugs etc.

My attempt to influence my reaction to the accident and its consequences was mostly embodied by the construction of the mental resilience reflex. I tried to be really responsible for my reaction to the indescribable difficulties I was dealing with. I decided not to hesitate and to resist stubbornly, time and time again, swiftly and with as little hesitation as possible. I often had to stop myself from brooding over my circumstances and forced myself to live from minute to minute. I was determined to do just about anything but crash.

This attitude is largely rooted in the personal observation that human behaviour is greatly determined by one's circumstances. Therefore, it is important to create a good, beneficial environment wherever possible. An organised approach for the long run seems to me the best 'free', 'conscious' and 'self-determined' way to live. For example, as a teacher in special-needs education, I have to organise well-advised and durable autism-friendly circumstances, as well as contribute to a positive and supportive atmosphere among colleagues. It works: people achieve higher and more complicated goals because of it. By working on certain long-term objectives in an organised way, it is possible to make a difference both daily and locally. Of course, the system is not infallible, 'the long term' can be a relative concept, and it takes thorough and continuous evaluation to make it work. In my case, a 'long time' can boil down to a couple of hours. Nonetheless, I have decided to compulsively make the most of the little time available to me in order to improve. Is this realistic and worth the denominator 'free will', or could we describe it more accurately as 'the specifically organised individual or collective will'?

On my 'quest for recovery', I stumbled upon an unexpected perspective in this regard.

In a series of articles in *Filosofie Magazine* (Hopster, 2015), free will sceptics Jeroen Hopster and Maarten Boudry argue it would be wrong to conclude that, in the absence of free will, no one is responsible for their own actions. Self-determination is not a prerequisite for responsibility; if anything, the opposite is true: we consider ourselves free because we can be held responsible. Hopster (building on the ideas of P.F. Strawson[15]) identifies a fallacy he calls 'overintellectualism': getting caught up in theories that undermine reality, when reality precedes that very same theory. First, there is the reality of us holding each other accountable, only then comes the notion that we act with free will – free will as a theoretical afterthought, if you will. This goes to show that profound theories and ideas can improve our understanding of reality, but also cloud it. If reality gets the better of a theory, then it is the theory that should be revised, not reality.

With the help of my wife, I would like to make the following addition: if society wasn't organised based on accountability, then the free will debate wouldn't have been an issue. Society, however, is in fact organised as such (consider, for instance, our justice system). Free will has as little to do with objective reality as concepts such as friendship, love and happiness: they are all vague concepts that we have to use to build something functional.

I won't go as far as to reject rational and empirical observations about free will in neuroscience because of this reason – indeed, they offer a more reliable view of reality – but the insight helps me to give the discussion a meaningful place in the way I deal with harsh reality. Moreover, it makes it easier to feel comfortable with a certain amount of pride in my resilience and willpower.

In sum (and at the risk of turning this into a semantic debate), I think the adjective 'free' does not fit with what we know about the observable phenomenon of will(power). However, with confidence in human reason and rationality, it seems possible nonetheless to direct the will in a long-term, organised way. Of course, this is a possibility and not a guarantee: much depends on the smallness of the scale and the nature of various circumstances.

So once again, when we apply this to my situation: I owe the fact I got this far in recovery to various circumstantial fortuities. Neurophysically, it is possible. I am well-surrounded by family and friends, I clearly have enough willpower and have managed to direct it through organisation and rationality. This is what I call 'the specifically organised will'. Maybe this aspect is best explained as a concrete, unique property of the human brain, acquired through natural selection.

This book became the thinking toolbox I used to organise, to *design*, my life and my recovery. It was a gradual process. I realised early on the importance of immediately writing down my experiences in order to preserve them. The observation, however, that it would also lead to deeper insights and higher yields for my efforts came as a surprise, the power of which I soon got to know and have fully exploited ever since. It allowed me to 'look at myself from a distance' and give direction to my will in the long run. This is yet another instance of 'cognitive distancing' through 'language against the impairment'.

The Two-edged Sword of Exact Science and the Power of Insignificance

In my situation, I was overwhelmingly confronted with severe circumstances and had little control over my own reaction to such an unjust and coincidental stroke of bad luck. I had to make sure the thought didn't keep me up at night. What did this entail philosophically? I became more and more aware of my own insignificance and that of humanity as a whole. The rise and development of exact science felt like a double-edged sword.

On the one hand, I am very grateful for medical, technological and scientific progress. The fact I was born into this era literally saved my life. Never before were humans so resistant against disease and death as they are today and it fills me with pride and awe to be able to witness it up close.

On the other hand, exact science has brought about a series of Copernican revolutions that has ousted man from the centre of existence. Copernicus himself banned us from the middle of the universe and 'creation': it is the sun, not the earth, around which our solar system revolves – which in turn is but one of many without any central role to play. We are only one species among many others and contemporary neuroscience eliminates the thought that Homo sapiens holds an elevated position by virtue of its unique self-determination. Moreover, although we have a gigantic impact on our ecosystem, that ecosystem in itself is stashed away in a tiny corner of the vast universe. The exclamation 'I am significant' sounds ever stranger to me. Power is per definition insignificant.

The previous analogy is based on a paradigm shift in three parts, made up by Freud: Copernicus – Darwin – Freud himself. In the 19th century, this was an image frequently used in different intellectual approaches to reality. I purposely left out Freud, because we now know he wasn't always operating from a truly scientific tradition. He constructed hypotheses of the unconscious mind unfit for falsification and built a continuously self-affirming illusion. In the end, his interpretation had little to do with reality, but became a clever field of study in and by itself. Unconscious processes play a major role in our mental housekeeping, that much is clear from neuroscience. Over time, however, Freud's approach became sloppy and good showmanship rather than actual science. Was he the first populist in humanities?

I had a conversation with John (a friend of my wife, an employee at Ghent Hospital and a cherished acquaintance of mine) about the advantages and drawbacks of science. I had come to admire its realisations and progress more and more and founded my way of looking at life largely on rational, empiric and falsifiable science. John was less keen on this idea and had some doubts in this regard.

John's main objection was that a society governed by science also entails a certain loss. According to him, the enormous authority of the scientific tradition deprives man of alternative tools to give meaning to (and to emotionally experience) daily reality. Professional therapeutic care, for instance, requires first and foremost a personal and human approach, and not only an impersonal, scientific interaction with 'the patient'.

For the most part, I understood his reasoning. It was the first elaborate confrontation in my recovery with a negative valuation of scientific progress – a humbling experience that put my own views in perspective.

Science and technology have saved my life and given me valuable insights about reality, but they do not provide an adequate answer to all human needs. To my mind, proper science doesn't pretend to do so either. It is an intellectual tradition that starts from 'not knowing', fallibility, controllability, replicability and falsifiability.

John also uses the generation of a vast number of 'pointless jobs' to make his point. In this respect, capitalism, science and technology together make things get out of hand. 'Imagine being a worker at a conveyor belt, or an employee at a low-cost airline, used as commodities without the job satisfaction of delivering meaningful products' was about the gist of his perspective.

I also used my view of science as an intellectual tradition starting from 'not knowing' as a catalyst to determine what is truly and realistically key for a meaningful life. As a matter of fact, this was my second catalyst, as my confrontation with extreme adversity had also contributed to this. The exceptionality of the situation had honed my insights.

I become increasingly aware that true meaning lies in smallness. It is possible to exert truly meaningful influence in small spaces and in short spans of time.

Science corroborates the idea of limitedness through the insight that we as a species (Homo sapiens) live on borrowed time on a tiny planet. The confrontation with my vulnerability only further confirms this perspective: it is truly 'now or never', 'here or nowhere', and that, to my mind and in my experience, is a useful, concrete, realistic and valuable perspective.

Notes

1 Blaise Pascal is a 17th-century French philosopher and mathematician (Clarke, 2015).

2 Ignaas Devisch is a Belgian professor of philosophy and ethics, working at Ghent University. He specialises in medical philosophy and was once a teacher of mine.

3 In Dutch, the expression goes as follows: 'Elk voordeel heeft zijn nadeel.' Johan Cruijff, however, rephrases it as follows: 'Elk voordeel heb zijn nadeel,' which is grammatically and phonetically incorrect. Johan Cruijff is

a football player famous for his remarkable (pseudo-)philosophical one-liners, pronounced with a thick accent.

4 In May 1968, a large-scale student demonstration and a general revolt shook France (and other countries, such as Belgium) to its core. It is generally considered to have been key in realising progressive social change at the time (Rubin, 2018).

5 Effective Altruism is a recent philosophical movement propagated by philosophers such as Peter Singer and William MacAskill. Its core tenet is that there is a moral obligation to spend at least some of our resources on alleviating suffering and improving the lives of sentient beings, as well as to do so in the most effective way possible. The goal is to allocate limited resources (money, volunteering, advocacy, career) to the most effective charities tackling those problems that have the largest scale, tractability and level of neglect. To this end, cause areas and organisations working on them are systematically screened independently using a scientific methodology. This is a response to the traditional way of going about charity, where the effectiveness of the charitable act is rarely looked into by people who want to do good (Anon., 2020).

6 Martha Nussbaum is a contemporary philosopher who advocates the moral relevance of emotions. She does so by demonstrating that emotions are not mere instincts, but that they do have rational and cognitive value. In addition to mere emotional impulses (hunger, for instance), there are also some emotions (grief, for instance) that are based on assumptions and interpretations of reality, and those can be rejected when proven to be unfounded (Cates, 2003).

7 The Stoic interpretation of happiness – as advocated by, for instance, Epictetus, an Ancient Greek writer – assumes that we are not unhappy because of events, but by our interpretation of them. We are not, for instance, disturbed by a punch in the face, but by the conviction that the humiliation and the pain are bad. Stoics believe that changing our perception of things generally regarded as negative by considering moral goodness the only thing worth calling 'good' will lead to happiness. This philosophy therefore strongly believes in the malleability of our emotions and, consequently, our own happiness (Baltzly, 2019).

8 Modern Stoicism is the contemporary practice of Stoic principles (see note 12), adapted through insights from (among others) Cognitive Behavioural Therapy to our present-day needs. The focus is mainly on the self-help principle rather than on the normative ethical framework from the Ancient Stoics: we should accept what is beyond our control, as worrying about it only does us harm, and we can do so by separating the actual event from its interpretation and the consequent emotion. A famous proponent of this philosophy, for instance, is Massimo Pigliucci.

9 Maarten Boudry is a philosopher of science and current holder of the Etienne Vermeersch (see note 16) Chair of Critical Thinking at Ghent University. His most recent book is 'Science Unlimited? On the Challenges of Scientism', co-edited with Massimo Pigliucci (Boudry, 2017). He published more than 40 papers in academic journals and several popular books in Dutch on critical thinking, illusions and moral progress. He advocates the use of scientific sources and methodologies to assess and steer contemporary global developments. As a believer in progress, he concludes

that, contrary to popular belief, several major positive evolutions (economic welfare, the fight against discrimination, …) have become better and better over the last few decades and will most likely continue to do so in the near future – exponentially so, even.

10 A Belgian philosopher working at Ghent University who has written (among others) on free will and the neurobiological basis for moral behaviour.

11 One of the most famous Belgian philosophers, best known for his defence of atheism, abortion and euthanasia. He passed away in 2019.

12 Johan Braeckman is a professor at Ghent University, a bioethicist and a sceptic.

13 Ico Maly is an associate professor at Tilburg University (The Netherlands). He teaches Digital Media & Politics, Digital Ethnography and Knowledge in the Digital World. As a writer, he has analysed and discussed political parties and convictions, as well as social topics such as diversity.

14 Steven Pinker is a Canadian-American researcher of psychology and cognitive science, focussing on (among others) language acquisition, emotions, rationality and the cognitive basis of morality. Like Maarten Boudry (see note 14), he is a believer in progress.

15 Strawson was a 20th-century British philosopher who (among others) studied determinism and moral responsibility. As a compatibilist, he believed that these two concepts are not mutually exclusive and that pragmatically, for social relationships to be possible, the assumption of free agency is justified (Coates, 2021).

References

Anon. (2020) Introduction to Effective Altruism. https://www.effectivealtruism.org/articles/introduction-to-effective-altruism/.

Baltzly, Dirk (2019) Stoicism, in Zalta, Edward N., *The Stanford Encyclopedia of Philosophy*, https://plato.stanford.edu/archives/spr2019/entries/stoicism/.

Boudry, Maarten (2015) *Illusies voor gevorderen: Of waarom waarheid altijd beter is.* Antwerp: Polis.

Boudry, Maarten and Pigliucci, Massimo (2017) *Science Unlimited? The Challenges of Scientism.* Chicago: The University of Chicago Press.

Cates, Diana Fritz (2003) Conceiving Emotions: Martha Nussbaum's 'Upheavals of Thought', *The Journal of Religious Ethics*, 31(2): 325–341.

Clarke, Desmond (2015) Blaise Pascal, in Zalta, Edward N., *The Stanford Encyclopedia of Philosophy.* https://plato.stanford.edu/archives/fall2015/entries/pascal/.

Coates, D. Justin and McKenna, Michael (2021) Compatibilism, in Zalta, Edward N., *The Stanford Encyclopedia of Philosophy.* https://plato.stanford.edu/entries/compatibilism/.

Dawkins, Richard and Wong, Yan (2017) *Het verhaal van onze voorouder: Een pelgrimstocht naar de oorsprong van het leven.* Amsterdam: Nieuw Amsterdam.

Devisch, Ignaas (2016) *Rusteloosheid: Pleidooi voor een mateloos leven.* Amsterdam: De Bezige Bij.

Hopster, Jeroen (2015) Denkfouten: Overintellectualiseren, *Filosofie Magazine*, 12. https://www.filosofie.nl/magazines/filosofie-magazine-12-2015/.

Rubin, Alissa J. (2018) May 1968: A Month of Revolution Pushed France Into the Modern World, *The New York Times*. https://www.nytimes.com/2018/05/05/world/europe/france-may-1968-revolution.html.

Schmid, Wilhelm (2005) Levenskunst: Het onvermijdelijke, *Filosofie Magazine*, 12. https://www.filosofie.nl/magazines/filosofie-magazine-02-2005/.

Chapter 5

Social Recovery

Resident of a Rehab Centre (K7)

During my stay at the therapeutic apartment, I had a surprising meeting. On one of my 'walks' through the corridors of K7, I came across a former teacher who was giving an interview to a camera crew (presumably about medical philosophy and ethics, his field of research at the time). I walked towards him and asked him: 'Are you Ignaas Devisch?' If my memory serves me right, he replied: 'Still am,' which I thought was funny, so we started chatting – although I did most of the talking, which must have been an atypical situation for a professor. It was nice seeing someone from the past at a time when I was still living in relative isolation from society and as such it was yet another beautiful and positive moment of my recovery. I was one step closer to normality. I recognised Ignaas and was able to correctly assess our connection. Despite the fact I wasn't physically able at that time to read his work, he reassured me of the functionality of my memory and the feasibility of many valuable goals in life. When later I got in touch with Ignaas online, he told me he often thought back to our meeting and congratulated me on my courageous and dignified attitude in accepting my fate. It made him realise how lucky he was in life. His acknowledgement made me feel warm inside and I decided to use it as one of the tools at my disposal for achieving my goals. We kept in touch online and he agreed to write the preface to this book.

Besides the commitment of my therapists and the occasional contact with the outside world, I got a lot of support from those sharing my fate. Many residents at the rehab centre also suffered from an ABI, from road traffic victims to people with cardiovascular disease: the causes were diverse, as were the degrees of severity. Everyone dealt with it their own way. Still, many of us had the feeling of being part of a community, of being in the same boat. The days were hard and the

DOI: 10.4324/9781003205142-6

challenges big, persevering and making progress was tough, and many had a rough time mentally, yet still, we somehow managed to cooperate. We supported each other and were there for one another, there was empathy and belonging, despite personal problems. Over time, I found out that extremely difficult circumstances naturally lead to strong friendships and with many of these people, I made a connection for life.

This book is also dedicated to Willem, Sybille, Merel, Tom, Conny, Jasmien, Greet, Lien, Jesse, Geert … It took me a while to establish contact with people other than my family and parents, but my fellow residents were the first ones I could do it with. Given the smoothness of our communication via social media, I think we'll manage to stay in touch. Our bond and our mutual understanding are profound and permanent.

In the autumn of 2017, I could stay home for the weekends. At the beginning of December, I was allowed to move back home and go back to the centre during the day for therapy. Things went on like this until the next summer. Returning home and seeing the frequency of the therapy sessions decrease was a fantastic evolution, but also one with mixed feelings. Letting go of the daily assistance, on the other hand, was confrontational and my renewed autonomy came with a lot of insecurity, anxiousness and unrest. This was the part of the journey where I was on my own – a reality check for my self-reliance. For many of my 'rehab buddies' and me, this was a moment of doubt. I once again realised how important it is to be surrounded by the right people.

Parents Will Be Parents

My parents were there for me and my family, every single day. During the first months, prospects weren't good and there was much uncertainty. Still, it didn't stop them from doing everything they could. It is thanks to them I didn't lose my faith in humanity – on the contrary.

My parents represent the difference a well-organised group of people can make. Evolutionarily speaking, this skill lies at the heart of our success as a species. For me personally, it means the difference between survival and a life worth living. Together with my wife's parents, they have made possible what the brain surgeon had predicted after the installation of the shunt: that I would be able to live a meaningful life …

Mum and dad have been on an incredible journey during my recovery. There was the constant worrying for my survival and later for how much exactly I would recover. At the same time, they had to be strong to support my wife and kids. I cannot imagine what a challenge it must have been mentally. They found solace with each other. Together with my family, they were my tower of strength, every single day.

Actually, I even got to know them better in this difficult period in our lives. I noticed I inherited my positive outlook from my dad and my perseverance from my mum. Thanks, mum and dad!

My Wife and Children

Everything I've said so far can be rephrased in superlatives where my family is concerned. It's hard to describe what it must have been like for children aged seven and 10 to see their father slip away into an almost vegetative state. For a long time, besides school, their lives largely consisted of hospital visits. When I was in the ICU, they could only briefly see their father, who was lying there hooked up to all these machines. Briefly holding my hand was the only option to be close to me. Sometimes, they could go to the day-care facility of Ghent Hospital while my wife and parents were with me for hours. There wasn't any real contact for a long time. It took years to restore it and it was hard to maintain it. The challenge was unfathomable and my daughters were forced to miss me a lot. I lived on a desert island of decreased consciousness and limited load capacity. I didn't even manage to partake in simple activities with the family, such as playing a game, singing a song or making music together. I couldn't keep up, there wasn't enough energy available. When finally, for the first time in many months, I could play with my children again, they had two big, radiant smiles on their faces. It was a massive achievement. My younger daughter had especially missed the 'rougher' games, such as 'the dragon game' and being thrown into the swimming pool. For months, I couldn't take my daughters to their hobbies because I wasn't allowed to drive. Family outings to playgrounds, amusement parks or parties were impossible as well. I felt so useless, as if I had let everyone down. I could count on a lot of understanding and support from my wife and parents, but I missed being a father.

My energy, so it seemed, was limited for good. I had to rely on my wife to help me be involved in the family. Without her, I simply couldn't partake in family activities. I had to call on her for help with practical and organisational affairs, such as paying bills, housekeeping, doctor's visits, following up on the kids' school life and hobbies … My wife and children gave me the structure to make the most of my limited energy and live a normal life again. The tables had turned: I was the one in need of care and my kids were the ones to provide it, along with their mother.

When I came back home for the weekend for the very first time, I had prepared dinner for my family in occupational therapy. This came as a very pleasant surprise to my wife and daughters. I had had to suppress my stress and agitation with great effort and with the support of the therapists, but the reward was completely worth it: a genuine family moment at last. For the first time, I got closer to my main objective: to be there for my family.

My wife and kids had to learn how to deal with the new situation. There was no more normal family life. For a long time, I could only be active for a couple of hours. The price of starting an activity with the children was that I had to lie down for the rest of the day and became completely unavailable – assuming I had the energy to start an activity with them in the first place. Whenever I had done something previously, either outside or inside the house, there was no energy left for them. The contrast with their energetic father before the accident was stark.

Surprisingly impressive as the results of my recovery may have been, in terms of my family life, I felt like I was making far too little progress. It became increasingly difficult to accept the contrast with the way things were before. It was one of the hardest aspects of my impairments and even talking to my wife about it was a challenge. Whenever the topic came up, I was engulfed by an uncontrollable cascade of emotions, ranging from powerlessness to unrest, emotional confrontation, disappointment and even guilt. Finding a solid, durable and valuable position in my family for my new identity turned out to be the biggest hurdle in my recovery. It was this very struggle that made the true dimensions of my impairments apparent. In all other situations, it was possible to set clear boundaries and make sacrifices to gain something valuable. This was not so in my interaction with my family. Even the smallest choices not to do something (such as assisting with their homework, making a biking trip, not being able to dust) felt like defeat and was a heavy burden to bear. It was hard in general to let go of predetermined goals, but at home, it felt like it was downright unacceptable. It would remain more or less so for the rest of our family life.

The strength with which my daughters showed me understanding and care in such a difficult situation was unbelievable. They still did well in school and didn't give up their hobbies – a huge relief for sure – all thanks to their own determination and the support of their mother.

As it turned out, my wife's employer allowed time off to care for a dependant and a flexible rearrangement of the work schedule. My wife's efforts go to show that extensive and carefully balanced care can make the difference in the long run to many people in difficult situations. It is a personal and societal investment with very high returns, and the way my wife went about it was life-changing and impressive to say the least.

My wife coordinated the care provided by my environment. Without her commitment, I wouldn't have gotten this far. As an illustration: by consistently administering eye-drops at regular intervals for a long time, she managed to save my left eye. Only someone with the determination and the perseverance like hers could be up to the task. It was one of the many sacrifices she made for me and throughout my ordeal she truly became my heroine forever. My love for her was reaffirmed time and time again.

Everyone needs a little luck in their lives and having met my wife and being married to her is my share of good fortune. I couldn't possibly imagine how anyone could handle the situation better than she has. She has given our children a solid and useful foundation in these difficult circumstances. She has saved our family from heavy traumas and psychological issues. There isn't a better organiser and educator in the whole world. She has been both the anchor of my children and the quality coordinator of my recovery – no unnecessary luxury, given the multitude of medical specialisations involved. She has been present at every consultation and has created the right circumstances at home for my recovery.

My family has lived through an emotional rollercoaster. It will take a lot of time to fully recover and it is likely that the outcomes of the accident will determine our thoughts and actions for a long time. By talking a lot and creating a caring atmosphere, we must try to steer the way we cope and to give recovery every possible chance. It is my absolute priority to seize the opportunity to contribute to this.

Musician in a Band

I realised that people want to belong to a group and that groups have an interest in working towards a durable common objective. One way to do so is to join a soccer team, but personally, I preferred joining a band, not least because you age with more dignity in that line of work. I hadn't stopped playing music with others since I was 16 and had been part of many line-ups. I played subsequently for 'Dorian GrEy', 'Suburban Lighthouse', 'Denham', 'Saint Patrick and the Blues Potatoes' and 'Stolen Ponies' – all illustrious (albeit underground) projects. At the time of the accident, I was fortunate enough to be a member of a wonderful ensemble called 'Les Cochons Sublimes' (The Magnificent Pigs). At the age of 40, I could say I had known true friendship, in part (and especially) thanks to my fellow band members.

But then disaster struck and my contribution to the band was promptly suspended. The 'Cochons' had known each other for years and in this dire situation, they showed me the true value of sincere friendship. The band played on, but also kept my old seat warm until the day I would return. They were among the first to visit me in hospital.

When after months I was finally able to play the bass again, it turned out I had forgotten all of our songs. I still remembered the position of the notes and chords on the instrument itself, though, as knowledge stored in deeper layers of my memory through many years of experience. Unsurprisingly so, maybe: after all, I hadn't been a member of the 'Cochons' for that long. It also had been a while before I was motorically able to play my instrument again. The muscles in my arms and fingers had to be rebuilt from scratch. The 'Cochons' wrote down all the songs for me and patiently rehearsed while I was working on my motor skills. They restored my position as a fully-fledged band member in what I only can describe as the best that a sense of 'us' has to offer.

Slowly but surely, I managed to recognise patterns in the structure of the music again and thus gradually abandoned the music sheets. My brain finally managed to generate steady 'thinking tracks' by actively making music. Sometimes, I had the feeling that some of the knowledge from before the accident was resurfacing, although it's hard to say whether this was really the case.

Playing music apparently stimulates the brain in a very unique way. While doing so, many different brain areas are active at the same time and complex neural networks are created all over the brain. Being a musician, it seems, is an unparalleled form of neurotherapy and as such has not only yielded profound friendships but has also contributed to my cognitive recovery. Despite my hearing impairment, my membership of 'Les Cochons

Sublimes' has proved incredibly profitable and I am proud to be a part of this wonderful group of people. Thank you, Diete Paternoster, Charles De Lange, Marc Vanlangendonck, Wouter Van Leeuwen, Dirk De Keyzer and Arie De Keyzer.

Being part of a musical collective again wasn't easy. In addition to my dysfunctional stimulus processing, there was the hearing impairment that complicated things. My left ear wasn't working at all and the right one needed a custom earplug to prevent further damage. This changed the way I experienced music and for a long time, I was doubtful whether being a musician could still be part of my new identity. Music had always been an important aspect of my life, but now, things were different. I hardly listened to the radio or my vinyl collection anymore, and even the subscription to a streaming service that I had received as a recovery gift was rarely made use of, much to my regret. The fear of incurring further damage and the need for a stimuli-poor environment were simply too big. I was always nervous when I was about to take part in rehearsals because I thought it would require a lot of energy. Still, I noticed early on that perseverance was key. After band practice, I always went home with more energy than before. There were various reasons for this: the friendship and support, music as a form of neurotherapy, the environment of the rehearsal space (the workshop of sculptor, fellow musician and my friend Dirk De Keyzer) … Even the playing itself seemed to work out just fine, much to my relief. The drummer, my 'soulmate in groove', assured me that my sense of musical orientation and rhythm were still there. Personally, I had the feeling that in spite of my diminished hearing, my focus had become more precise. I lost myself in the music in a completely new fashion. I was so glad I could be a part of all this again that I rediscovered how much I loved to dance: I couldn't keep my feet still for the entirety of the rehearsals or shows. It was my way of celebrating my regained mobility and standing up and moving became an inexhaustible source of joy. I jokingly called myself 'the only folk bass player who can't stop dancing'. In my dreams, it became my new trademark. There should be room for a quip every now and then …

Performing with the 'Cochons' was one of the first steps in the outside world and it turned out to be a source of joy and energy. The warm reception of the audience gave me just the extra support I needed for my well-being. I practised a lot to make it happen. The first time, I only joined for five songs. I continuously worked on extending my participation. However, some elements of being a musician were lost for the most part. I went to band practice and took part in shows, but afterwards I went straight back home. The limit to my available energy forced me to set clear boundaries and stick to them.

Restart 2.0: Meaningful Work for Experts by Experience

One of the biggest motivators throughout recovery was the prospect of getting back to work. I expressed my motivation in the following 'tested expression': 'I truly have meaningful work for which I got a lot of appreciation in return from pupils and colleagues. I miss it and I want it back.'

I know from experience that the way my school operates (Campus Impuls – Reynaertschool, GO! Ghent) can make a difference to a great number of pupils. Because of our work, both the youngsters themselves and their immediate surroundings can profit from the pupils' search for meaningful participation in society.

Working at a school for people with an autism spectrum disorder (ASD) and both normally and highly intellectually gifted youngsters is the epitome of meaningful work. We adapt to the requirements that come with ASD: smaller groups, more structure and predictability, paramedical support from psychologists and the remedial education team, ... Watching our pupils find the emotional rest they need to seize the opportunities we provide them with is the most touching experience I have ever had in my life. This is what meaningful work truly can achieve.

A prime example that I'll never forget is the story of Rupert Cardyn. When Rupert first came to our school, he was going through an emotionally turbulent time. He constantly isolated himself and lacked the confidence and the structure to establish meaningful contact with those around him. He had lost faith in himself and others after a series of negative social experiences and due to acute overstimulation. Rupert, like all of our students, was given the diagnosis of ASD and his specific way of thinking lied at the heart of the distance between himself and his surroundings. At first, the situation seemed hopeless, but in the end, thanks to the elaborate autism-friendly adaptations that were put in place, things took a turn for the better. After several months, his perseverance prevailed. It soon became clear that Rupert had a great sense of justice, which we encouraged and focussed on together so that through his motivation, he made it his life's mission to help those in vulnerable positions. After a few years, he became a school representative and even a Flemish representative in Brazil for YOUCA (Youth for

Change and Action[1]) in 2016. As such, he was given the opportunity to travel around the world to fulfil his ambitions, which was a huge boost for his self-perception. I have witnessed first-hand how he learned to enjoy life – an unforgettable experience.

A couple of months before my own accident, Rupert, aged 17 at the time, died in a traffic accident. He was hit by a car while riding on his bike. I will never forget him. I dedicate the second chance I got in life to him.

The prospect of getting back to work got me all fired-up. I started riding my bike to work again (9 km) and overcame the fears I had come to associate with it. I practiced keeping my balance and my coordination extra hard and even bought a new bike for the occasion.

I had been given some theoretical information about the consequences of an ABI at the rehab centre. It struck me that, besides the many differences, there were also quite some similarities with ASD. The most striking ones were:

- dysfunctional stimulus processing;
- overchoice;
- problems using executive (i.e. problem-solving and controlling) cognitive functions at unexpected moments;
- somewhat weaker time management skills and extra sensitivity to time pressure;
- orientation problems (time and space).

'Tested expression': 'From now on, I'll be able to speak from experience when standing in front of classes with an ASD focus.'

Oftentimes I found myself at a loss in front of the wardrobe, unable to decide on what I would wear that day. Beautiful weather posed a dilemma: linen shorts or jeans? Under normal circumstances, this used to be an easy choice, but now it had become a sensitive situation. It stressed me out, especially as the clock was ticking – at least in my head: there was little rational reason for feeling pressed for time. It was only a matter of seconds, in the worst case a matter of minutes, in no way something that would endanger the remainder of my schedule, but still, it felt like it would.

An important aspect of my recovery was swimming laps, which at a certain point I did in the Olympic pool called 'Rozebroeken' in Ghent. Here, I always picked lane 7, because doing so was the only way to avoid anxiousness. There was no logic to it: it just so happened that the first time I had swum in this pool, I had done so in lane 7.

Encountering unexpected problems during daily activities brought about more problems than it used to. During the first days at work, I took on an additional chore: making name plates for the school, which to me seemed easy enough. It involved saving some files on a flash drive. At a certain point, however, I noticed I had lost the folder in which I had stored these files. I started swearing and completely shut down. My wife had to help retrieve everything and for a moment, I was at a loss and couldn't function anymore – a clear indication that I was still held back by my impairments. It came as a blow. So despite the many differences between an ABI and ASD, I mostly experienced the similarities.

I felt forced to tread carefully and act prudently if I wanted my return to work to succeed. As a long-distance runner, I had already learned to set my pace wisely and to stay within the boundaries of my abilities. I needed to apply this knowledge to other situations as well, especially to my job. Luckily, by then I had learned to transfer skills from one situation to another – a difference with many (but not all) people with ASD.

It is important to note, however, that there are a lot of differences within the group of people with an ABI or with ASD. Every individual shows some level of variation amidst a set of common characteristics.

Gradually regaining my independence became an ever-growing part of my personal recovery. Where once I used to be a rather chaotic person, I now was forced to structure things more meticulously. Therefore, as soon as I could read and write again, I had a computer to categorise all work- and recovery-related information with. I also had the ambition to cover all aspects of the non-confessional ethics curriculum in the last two years of high school. I didn't want any more holes in my course material, which was complicated by the fact that I predominantly used to work with the Socratic method and expected a lot of input from my pupils. My need for structure and predictability often got the upper hand and largely governed my actions.

In September 2018, the time had finally come: I could get back to work as part of my 'recovery continued on the work floor' – an initiative by the rehabilitation centre. At the time, it hadn't been around for long. As such, it was completely unknown to my school, who consequently weren't expecting this at all. Officially, I was still on sick leave and had a full-time replacement. I was very lucky that the headmistress and the support team of coordinators decided to take a calculated risk and give me and the program a chance. Marijke, Arne and Tom did their utmost to make the most of it and the importance of their decision for my mental wellbeing cannot be understated. It was finally happening!

At first, I worked four hours a week. This wasn't much for someone who used to be a full-time teacher, so given my eagerness to be fully involved as a part of the school and its staff again, I had a hard time accepting those conditions. It was important for my self-worth to get as close to normal life as possible. Then again, having enough energy to perform useful labour was key for that ambition. I could count on the well-advised assessment of the centre's neuropsychologist and doctor to soundly start working again and so I took their advice to start with four hours – a realistic choice that saved me from relapse due to overexertion and stress.

I had to prove in this situation that I was still a rational thinker. I had to acknowledge that a slow, gradual restart would be the best approach. It soon became clear that I wouldn't need any theoretical reason to be convinced of the fact: in reality, there simply wasn't any worthy (let alone a better) alternative. This I came to know through experience. The start of a new term always involves a lot of work and the fact our school was moving to another building at the time added to that. I helped out wherever I could and attended parent-teacher conferences and staff meetings. It didn't take long before I exceeded the four-hour limit …

The first real class I taught was on Tuesday, September 4. I was elated and stressed at the same time. I hadn't taught in one year and four months and the anticipation of this moment amounted to a cocktail of high hopes and nagging insecurity. The outcome wasn't bad per se, but it could have been better. I was still too often the one to do the talking. The night after my first class, I was overcome by fatigue and craved a stimuli-poor environment, which motivated me to go to bed at 18:30. I didn't have any trouble falling asleep that evening and woke up at 09:30 the next morning. I hadn't had to retreat to stimuli-free places since my time at the rehab centre. Back then, it had been a habit for many weeks, but that was already months ago. My first day at work made it crystal-clear that I had to take things easy, especially under heavy workloads. Luckily, I was no stranger to this sort of situation and by now I had the experience necessary to adapt my behaviour and expectations accordingly. Still, I was given yet another reminder at the end of that same week. I had been aiming for 10 km more regularly during my 'glorified speed-walking' practice. When I tried to make it the first week of September 2018, I couldn't manage to keep my heartbeat in check and consequently had to shorten the distance and lower the speed. My body showed me once again that in terms of energy, balancing supply and demand remained a delicate affair and that I couldn't afford to overdo it. Energy consumed for work couldn't be used for any other purpose anymore: there was simply no surplus.

Taking things easy immediately paid off. My second class, two days later, was a success. I knew from a rehearsal at the rehab centre some months prior that I could still do it and this class was the ultimate confirmation of that impression. I realised how much I enjoyed doing this, which only went to show that the essence of my personality was still intact, that the brain injury hadn't erased my true nature. Mr. Geerinck had survived and still very much enjoyed what he was doing.

The subjects of the second class were:

- is it possible not to think?
- are dark thoughts always a bad thing?
- do dark thoughts serve any purpose?
- is the meaning of life different for everyone?
- is phantasy a form of thinking?
- is day-dreaming a form of thinking?

We had a truly meaningful conversation about these subjects, 'thinking about thinking' as it were, and the pupils visibly enjoyed it. Getting this close to the essence of my job so early in the resumption of my work gave me a great mental boost.

Taking things slowly was key, but even so, I couldn't resist the urge to get involved in a workshop called 'musical band'.

Our school also tries to help its pupils develop meaningful pastimes. To this end, I am the co-founder of a workshop called 'musical band'. It is one of the realisations that I am most proud of professionally and I thoroughly enjoy these magical moments of youngsters making music together. It is truly a form of brain training with a big social aspect to it.

Taking up this part of the job right from the start was not without its risks. I could cross my boundaries, something I tried to avoid at all costs. Still, the prospect of all the satisfaction it would give me was too tempting, so I went ahead anyway, with the precaution of using the hearing protection to avoid further damage to my right ear. My calculated risk immediately paid off: I got a lot of job satisfaction and gratitude from pupils and colleagues in return. It was a decision that came with a lot of anxiety, but it was completely worth it.

Returning to work was a major step towards normality and it felt like true, demonstrable progress. I soon noticed, however, that progress doesn't necessarily mean that things get easier. I was forced to kick-start daily life myself, which required an enormous adaptation on my part. I had to continuously convince myself that if it were to happen, it had to be on a day-to-day basis. Every morning I struggled to finish what I used to do almost automatically before. The first weeks, I was already visibly tired after getting up, having breakfast, getting dressed, preparing my bag and closing the front door behind me. The day was yet to start. This weighed heavily on my morale. Then again, it helped to focus on the reason I was doing all of this: optimism had become a moral duty, something I owed both to myself and my family. This realisation grew in significance amidst these new and challenging circumstances.

Triple Booking and Energy Deficit: Justice, Work and Surgery

The first phase of resuming work lasted for three weeks and coincided with court case preparations and the facial surgery that took 11 hours. I would be off on sick leave for six weeks, unable to work or do sport. Moreover, the day after surgery, the first court hearing of my accident would take place. It was pretty much a lost case for the defendant: she had had 1.98 per ml of alcohol in her blood when she ran me over – in other words: she had been absolutely wasted. An eyewitness had declared that she had been swaying left and right for a while prior to the collision. Moreover, an expert opinion confirmed I had been riding on the bicycle path and that it had been impossible for me to avoid the accident. In short, there was little room for doubt, but still, the verdict hadn't been passed yet and I really needed one to claim financial compensation. The defence tried to get out of paying by pleading 'intoxication' rather than 'drunkenness',[2] which, if the plea would be accepted, would prevent the driver's insurance company from claiming any money from her personally. I cared little about the semantics: all I needed was a written acknowledgement of indisputable and full liability. The defence didn't contest this, but for some procedural reason they postponed admittance and thus delayed the case.

All the uncertainties this juridical battle entailed didn't make recovering easier. I wanted to be financially independent, as was my right. My faith in justice – which to my mind was also part of a meaningful life – was on the line. I held on to the ambition to get back to working full-time, but I needed the reassurance that I wouldn't get into trouble financially if it didn't pan out. All I could do was wait for the judge's verdict.

It was hard to distribute my energy and loads wisely at this stage. I wanted to be physically strong in preparation for the complicated surgery of my face and aimed more often for running 10 km. I managed more and more often to cover that distance in a responsible way. I forced myself to stay within the limits of an acceptable heart rate and not to cross any boundaries that would set me back. Out of the five registered running trails, I stubbornly stuck to trail three – a scenic, safe and green route.

I noticed that by resuming work, I consumed more energy. Since my energy supply was still significantly lower than it used to be, this had its impact on my physical recovery. For weeks on end, I had trouble keeping my heart beat low, so I had to shorten the distance and lower the pace. I had just managed to turn 'glorified speed-walking' into running, but now once again had to let go of that achievement. As far as speed was concerned, I could not but hold back. In preparation for the surgery, however, I worked hard to be able to cover 10 km again. I had been prioritising distance over pace for a while at the time, so I was ok with this trade-off. Still, it once again became clear that recovery is not a straight upward slope, but a continuous cycle of progress and relapse.

The multitude of impressions and the growing activity of the days once again gave me no choice but to live from day to day, sometimes even from hour to hour. The pressure was of such proportions that thinking about the following day or even the upcoming afternoon was pointless. At times, the stream of thoughts was unstoppable and again, it was my sleep that was affected most because of it. I lay awake for hours, with nothing but my hyperactive consciousness to keep me company.

The week before surgery and the court case was the worst in this respect. First, there was the anxiety for the upcoming operation. Despite my worries, I had to focus on the last classes in the first phase of my return to work, which was further complicated by the presence of a film crew who were there to shoot a documentary on facial surgery. Then there were two parties for family and friends that were scheduled for that week and an appointment with my lawyer. I had to focus mentally to distance myself from this multitude of events and not to drown in my counterproductively dark thoughts. I had to use all available energy and willpower. Giving up after getting this far simply wasn't an option.

In the end, I succeeded by introducing stimuli-poor breaks into my daily schedule and by carefully pacing myself.

Notes

1 A Belgian organisation that encourages youngsters to help create a more sustainable and fairer world by raising awareness and supporting both domestic and international projects.

2 A juridical distinction based on the amount of alcohol detected in the blood, but of little relevance for this particular court case given that the driver by far exceeded the limits of either category.

Chapter 6

Financial Recovery

Impersonality in a Contemporary System of Anonymous Solidarity: Justice in a Complex Society

The biggest mental hurdle was yet to come …

> Sometimes it seems almost impossible to constructively process emotions. The harder the circumstances, the bigger the challenge. What follows is the story of one of the most difficult moments of my life in this respect.
>
> In my book, I write about the fight against anxiety in traffic, against the fear of epilepsy, against depressed feelings and counterproductive rancour. This chapter is about strong, compulsive feelings of injustice and the attempt to deal with them rationally. I have spent enormous amounts of energy trying to transform my experiences and perceptions into a workable and constructive reaction. It took a lot of time and thought, but in the end, I pulled it off.

The aforementioned court case had come to a close: the judge had found the drunk driver guilty of the accident beyond a reasonable doubt. This was the verdict I needed to recover my sick days, which in turn would allow me to secure my claim to financial compensation. My employer (the Flemish Community[1]) would then be able to claim for expenses on the insurance policy of the driver. In case of a 'non-work-related injury', a verdict of full liability is a prerequisite for long-term indemnification as per the law of Belgium. At least, that is what they told me.

In the end, the verdict proved not to be sufficient in itself. As long as the insurance company decided to postpone payment (which of course they did, because the calculations of all costs had not been finalised

DOI: 10.4324/9781003205142-7

yet), so too would the Flemish Community. In the meantime, my sick days were depleted, which meant that my salary was reduced, regardless of the verdict. In other words: as long as the insurance company didn't pay up, the Flemish Community basically said 'no deal' to me. I was on my own, with 59% of my original salary. This led to the harsh (and hopefully premature) conclusion that the society to which I belonged insufficiently subscribed to moral justice. So too, to my mind, did the procedures and laws that were supposed to guarantee anonymous solidarity in this country. All that mattered in the end was cold, hard cash. The fact I had to maintain a family and pay my mortgage apparently was my problem and mine alone – hence my emotional reaction that it is my absolute priority to be there for my family and to protect them from the long-term negative consequences of what was in essence nothing but a stroke of misfortune. I did not want to put my wife and daughters in a situation of financial insecurity. I saw it as the duty of society to protect me and that it should claim on the insurance policy afterwards, regardless of my trajectory. After all, I was the one in the right.

The system of solidarity in our community, to my mind, had outrageously failed me. I had fought so hard to get where I was and was dealt a shamelessly heavy blow where I least expected it – such was my first emotional reaction. It proved to be an unworkable one and it persisted no matter what.

My patience was seriously tested and I considered quitting the current trajectory of my recovery and going back to full-time employment, effective immediately, against the advice of the therapists. It was my job, my place in the school community, my meaningful work, and I would have it no other way! If I couldn't count on society's solidarity, then I would make it on my own. This too I could do, here too I would move boundaries without crossing them and crashing. I was the one in charge of my life, not some insurance company or the Flemish Community. I had made it this far and I would make it even further, they'll see. If they would force me to, I would instantly become the whistleblower of this manifest injustice to as large an audience as possible.

The anger and thirst for vengeance were hard to redirect into a constructive direction. In my thoughts, I was brooding on a plan. I already had a documentary, a book that was being written and verbal skills honed by the demanding circumstances of my physical impairment. I would launch a media campaign. It was the conversations with my wife that calmed me down and convinced me to wait a little longer. My urges and thoughts needed restraint, and restraint they found in the care of smart people around me.

The Flemish Community's mission in this regard, so they maintained, was to be a reliable mediator between policy and practice and a partner in the development and execution of the former. As far as the development and execution of the policy was concerned, I had expected a human touch that went beyond mere money-driven arguments. As to their so-called 'reliability' as a partner, I felt ashamed on their behalf. According to my fearful interpretation at the time, they kept urging me to have false faith in allegedly 'binding' procedures, but when it came to hard cash, these rules meant nothing. I was dropped like a hot brick and all the benefits I had so faithfully contributed to society over the years didn't seem to matter much. I had always willingly paid my taxes without complaining because I knew the value of social security and the general good as such, but now that I needed to rely on its services, I was at the mercy of a private insurance company. It all seemed so toxic, so pointless, so outdated.

I know that in our modern, complex society, a personal and informal approach to solidarity is no longer practically feasible. It takes general rules and procedures to ensure justice and solidarity. A prerequisite for finding that acceptable, however, is that these rules and procedures start from the needs of the most vulnerable social groups and are applied accordingly.

In this respect also, the government failed me, the realisation of which was hard to process. It defies belief, especially for someone with an ABI and a diminished load capacity. I was under the impression that our country's executive power had degenerated into an endless, pointless administration, where laws were replaced by informal and random deals. The spectre of bureaucracy was haunting my world and I could only hope my attempts to get the better of it via my lawyer would be successful eventually, without negative effects on the remainder of my journey. I feared there would be no justice to be found for me if the interpretation of the law was this prone to randomness. The civil servants of the relevant agency, moreover, struck me as chronically slow and subservient to the senseless automation of bureaucracy. I had seemingly wound up in a Kafkaesque tragedy and could only hope for a favourable outcome. Fortunately, there was light at the end of the tunnel and as it soon would turn out, there was also reason to be positive about the way my case was concluded in the end.

I want to stress that I do not hold the civil servants of the agency responsible and that I do not hold a grudge against either them or society as a whole. As I said before, I want to bring a positive story and I derive more energy from a positive perspective on what happened. That does not mean, however, that I won't point out the things I find unacceptable with the intent of improving society. Maybe some conclusions can be drawn from my experience that will help the public departments involved to become more effective. With the cards I've been dealt, I want to create something valuable for myself, others and society as a whole. I don't have another choice. It feels like a moral imperative. As a citizen, I want nothing more and nothing less than a reliable legal framework.

At a certain moment, I had the feeling I was losing control of the situation. To be sure, my lawyer did everything he could to defend my rights, and so did the government, if we're being honest; there were two juridical services working in my best interest. The risk, however, was that they would work against each other, as they both abided by a different interpretation of the law. The government agency went by the procedure they always used in case of a non-work-related injury. My lawyer maintained this was in conflict with the law that was referred to. I decided to call all parties involved, insisted on an amicable settlement and asked them to dovetail their approaches. I showed my appreciation for the agency's efforts to remind the insurance company of its duties and stressed that I wanted to avoid or reverse any potential conflict. All the while, I was drawing on a tactic I used as a teacher and that I derived from the 'New Authority' concept:[2] to react only when the initial anger has subsided. Funnelling my emotionality into this effort was a way of turning a challenging situation into a meaningful contribution. Eventually, the agency handed a written argument to my lawyer, who promised me he wouldn't undertake anything without consulting me first. I had taken matters into my own hands again and it felt like victory over my presumed impairments.

I realised that maybe it's somewhat of an emotional reaction and even a slight exaggeration, but the way I saw it, the imaginary order of the 'Flemish Community' lost all of its credibility in these precarious times. It seemed nothing more than an illusion that couldn't meet the conditions of its own existence. 'Flanders' to me instantly ceased to exist. The situation made a laughingstock of the entire construct and it had no longer something useful to contribute to the reconstruction of my identity. I instantly felt stateless, Belgian and Flemish in name only for the sake of worldly, administrative recognition, but bereft of any connection to the underlying fantasy. I had become a citizen of the world, a homeless individual, surviving in spite of my nationality on paper, relying on my own strength. I had already been sympathetic to the notion of cosmopolitanism before and it fitted well with my personality and convictions, but now this sentiment was firmly amplified.

My emotional reaction was intense, but it also had a rational basis. The moral principles at the heart of my attitude in life were violated. To my mind, the unexpected turn of events that instantly had made me a fragile individual accurately exemplified the importance of the following ethical paradigm:

> We all live in a reality veiled in uncertainty. Nobody knows their fate within the next week, month or year. National institutions with high levels of welfare should use this realisation to protect the most vulnerable in their society. Of course, there is room for luxury and differences in welfare, but only when the wellbeing of those most at risk has been safeguarded. It's a political and moral thought experiment devised by John Rawls, but sometimes also becomes a bitter reality, as illustrated by my case.

I could only conclude that my own Western-European welfare state still left an awful lot to be desired and should urgently get its priorities straight. Professionals from the medical sector said they knew from experience that oftentimes, people in need of care have to wait for the means which they are legally entitled to. Safe to say that there was room for significant improvement: my society wasn't just, fair or reasonable enough yet …

Inspired by the work of a former fellow-student, Ico Maly, the situation led me to a strong conclusion: it seemed of the utmost importance to defend ideas of equality and basic rights for all in our globalised world, especially for those of us who are dealt a bad hand. In our present-day context, this needs to be enacted on a supranational scale. I felt even more sympathetic to the core ideals of Enlightenment (radical as they were at the time) than before.

> The world can be, and has to be, more just. Everyone is born with the same natural rights. Hence, not only do immigrants have duties, but also inalienable rights, as do people who require extra care. If, like in my case, these rights are not automatically safeguarded or if they are subjected to random interpretation, this only makes matters worse for those people. In my case, liability was legally well-defined and the defence well-insured, so there was

no room for doubt and I should have received the support I needed. Here too I do not merely reason from a rational, empathetic or professional point of view, but also from personal experience with reliance on care. The right to social security doesn't seem to be adequately developed and cannot be sufficiently invoked yet, despite the fact that we are better than we've ever been in this respect. There is room for improvement, if only we are willing to seize the opportunity.

The existing legal framework, juridically determined liability and the efforts of my own lawyer and those of the responsible government agency ultimately saved me from excessively negative consequences. The system, in other words, had laid the foundations of an acceptable outcome, even though two years later, the actual outcome was yet undetermined.

It was safe to assume that everyone involved acted in good faith to the best of their abilities. I sincerely thanked the employee of the agency over the phone for her help in my search for a just resolution.

What, then, can we conclude?

It turns out that ideas and procedures that underpin a just societal system must be continuously monitored and corrected. The rights of those in vulnerable positions easily erode in bureaucratic systems. Without the vigilance of juridical experts, civil-society organisations, politicians, competent civil servants or interest groups, legally protected rights may fall victim to random interpretation and so become prone to injustice.

Every system is susceptible to abuse and unexpected perverse effects. As it would be naive to assume that everyone calling on social services for help has noble intentions, a stable, just and consistent system requires a strong judge. Still, solidarity and vigilance are not opposites.

Last but not least: we are richer than we've ever been before and our current level of welfare and wellbeing exceeds anything we've seen before by far. The empirical and scientific evidence that supports this is enormous. We therefore have the unique opportunity to help a tremendous number of people, which is what we're doing already, of course, but with the right means and methods, we can do even more. This is in our own interest as well as in that of others, a mutually beneficial expression of one of our most impressive human abilities: to cooperate on a large scale in incredibly challenging and complicated circumstances.

Luckily, my character prevented me from getting depressed or holding a grudge, as did my lack of energy and the realisation that such negative feelings would only be counterproductive. I was reminded of what deep disappointment felt like: a stark contrast with all things meaningful in life, which, luckily, were still in ample supply. Eventually, there seemed to be a lasting and acceptable solution as a result of the good will and open communication of all involved. The latter in particular had proven to be fragile and had required a lot of investment from me as a citizen. It goes to show the importance of investing as a society in durable communication within a reliable juridical system.

Notes

1 The government institution in the northern part of Belgium (Flanders), in charge of (among others) education.

2 A model for parents and educators to resist (self-)destructive behaviour of children. It is based on non-violent resistance and was founded by Professor Haim Omer (Omer, 2010).

Reference

Omer, Haim (2010) *The New Authority: Family, School and Community.* Cambridge: Cambridge University Press.

Chapter 7

Two Years and Counting

The Moment of Truth: The Importance of the Second Year

As 2018 turned into 2019, I managed to stay up until midnight on New Year's Eve. Watching my children and their friends count down and party brought tears to my eyes. The fact I could be a part of it all at such a symbolic time was simply overwhelming. Still, it would be a demanding year: my optimism would be put to the test by the many compulsory doctor consultations, the court case would come to an end, the degree of my invalidity would finally be determined, the resumption of my work would enter a new, decisive phase and the reanimation of the left part of my face was due nine months after the nerve had been implanted. The reconstruction of my existence was next on the agenda.

Still, I faced new and dynamic challenges in making out the degree of my impairment on the one hand and determining what was truly possible on the other. My possibilities had increased, but the feasibility of my aspirations often collided with reality. My optimism, willpower and confidence had to remain realistic – a challenging task in and by itself. I had demonstrated in the course of my recovery that hope can be self-fulfilling and believing in myself had turned out to be really rewarding. Still, I couldn't afford to give in to hubris. I had to assess the demanding circumstances and my abilities accurately. My body had proven its resilience, partly thanks to the nature of the injuries, that allowed for a reasonable degree of recovery, and also thanks to my good physical condition at the time of the accident. I had become a specialist in careful recovery, but that didn't mean there was no further need for me to stay sharp and get even better. I hadn't crossed the finishing line yet and I started to realise that I would have to keep this up for the rest of my life. My ambition to get as close to normality as

DOI: 10.4324/9781003205142-8

possible hadn't changed, but the chronic and difficult nature of the circumstances was weighing heavily on me. The inverse proportionality that came with favourable evolutions only added to this impression: the closer I got to my former self, the harder the nagging feelings of doubt became. Yes, what I had built thus far approximated a normal life, which made me happy, but would I truly be able to be a fully-fledged member of society again, to fulfil my aspiration of making a difference? The truth was there would be no finishing line, and my desire for it had been the pitfall my therapists kept warning me about and that I experienced more and more. Belief in a happy ending isn't always self-fulfilling, as I had found out both mentally and physically (thanks to Maarten Boudry (2015)'Illusies voor gevorderden' ('An Advanced Guide to Illusions') for the theoretical wake-up call). In sum: to a large extent, my injuries and their collateral damage were for life.

The struggle would go on, that much was sure, but the question became: on which level, broadly speaking? Many therapists and doctors – from the physical therapist the first months after the accident to the principal doctor at K7 – had told me throughout my recovery that the first two years would be decisive. The progress I would have made by then would be a good indication of what would be feasible altogether. This is not to say that there would be no further evolution after two years, but for the most part, the broad outlines of what was still possible would have been set out by then. It would be the moment of truth: to what degree had I preserved my identity and how much would I inevitably have to concede to my impairment? What could be a meaningful way of living my life for me, my wife, my children and everyone else around me? Would recovery not only increase its reach, but also get easier and fall within the limits of normality more consistently? Was returning to an average and controllable life realistic? For recovering patients, this was a common point of reference and likewise, it was somewhat of a deadline for the medical examiner, who was to determine my degree of invalidity to calculate the compensation from the insurance policy of the driver. For me too, the moment had evolved into a symbolic date with a lot of potential, something to work up to ever more intensely. It would be an emotional moment, especially now that I had been finally able to shift from a relentless fighting mode to a more sensitive and reflective approach to my second life. This seemed to me the perfect opportunity to finish this book completely and move on.

As the Smoke Clears: Life after Recovery

I was constantly caught between two conflicting observations. On the one hand, I remembered my former self well and recognised big parts of it in my new situation. On the other hand, my physical appearance and mental balance had changed tremendously. The daily confrontation with reality's demands led to feelings of stagnation and relapse. No aspect of life was self-evident anymore. The search for more possibilities and the desire for progress required a daily functional reset of my perseverance. The feeling of having to start from nothing every single morning was a given. Every day was a blank page that had to be written all over again. I couldn't fall back on achievements of the past month, week or even day. This meant that satisfaction and contentment could only be derived from present realisations, which led me to put enormous pressure on myself. The bar was raised high, as was demanded by the complexity of my recovery, which simply didn't allow me to rest on my laurels – indeed, there weren't any to begin with as soon as the sun rose. Getting back to a normal life would henceforth mean working hard 24/7, for the rest of my life. I continuously had to balance out negative mental perceptions of my impairment and come to terms with what would be the definitive version of normality from now on. The brain injury and the bodily damage would henceforth shape the remainder of my life, incessantly and relentlessly. Just how much it would do so, as mentioned before, gradually became clear in the second year after the accident.

At the beginning of February 2019, I attended the second annual memorial service of Rupert Cardyn at our school. He would forever be 17.

> The parallels between his story and mine (a traffic accident while on a bike, only in his case with a deadly outcome) truly touch me and will forever play an important role in my second life. Rupert and I got along well and the similarity of our ill fortune only further adds to my connection with him and what he has left behind. His commitment and his sincere pursuit of justice will always be a source of inspiration to me personally as well as to our school community. Rupert has made a difference: his life was truly meaningful.

There came the tears again. The journey so far had definitely taken a heavy toll on my feelings. For the second time, I involuntarily visualised the many scars on my body and went through the emotional rollercoaster of the past one and a half years. It had been two years since Rupert had left us and it would soon be two years since my very own accident. The coincidence overwhelmed me. His father and mother were present too. Once a silver birch was planted in his memory and after a rendition of 'The Sound of Silence' by two pupils of our school's band, his mum and I found ourselves embracing each other as a confirmation of our permanent connectedness – yet another realisation of her son.

And then came the first meeting with the medical examiner appointed by the court at the beginning of February. It went more smoothly than I had anticipated. I had been very stressed in advance, but the conversation turned out to be fair. I was accompanied by Doctor Oostra of Ghent Hospital and the other doctors present (those of a 'neutral third party' and those of the defence) were impressed with the extensiveness of my case. A real medical examination was yet to be performed and given that my situation was considered to be still evolving, they wished to see me again at the end of 2019. No definitive conclusions would be drawn until then. I hadn't expected otherwise. For now, however, the feeling of being treated fairly was an important observation that gave me great peace of mind. And, what was more: even though my situation was considered to be still evolving, the broad outlines of the permanent damage would nonetheless become clearer and clearer in the upcoming year. Recovery was largely over; the struggle, on the other hand, was not, but at least now life truly could begin again.

The week after the meeting with the medical examiner, I had a follow-up consultation with the neurosurgeon. I felt the tension rise in my body but managed to stay relatively calm in anticipation of the moment. The most recent scans were scrutinised and the position and condition of my shunt were verified. There were no indications of additional complications. The shunt was still in its correct position and there were no signs of recent epileptic activity in the scans. It seemed that the brain damage was under control and that significant improvements were being made. I wouldn't have to abandon hope of a normal life! The realisation cleared a lot of space in my brain. I left the hospital with a broad (albeit half-sided) grin and felt a stream of new energy that I used to take on extra work at home. I had long conversations with my children and vacuum-cleaned forgotten corners, just because I could.

The final round of facial surgery was scheduled for the end of February. It was to be a minor operation, but it would nonetheless be the ninth time I was fully anaesthetised. The surgery had had to take place in multiple rounds because it had been hard to predict how the transplanted fat tissue would react, so there was still some 'touching-up' to be done (that's what the doctors called it, I didn't make it up myself). It was the first time after a surgery that I could get dressed all by myself, walk to the car and drive back home to sleep in my own bed. The difference the intervention made socially was significant to say the least: over time, people stopped treating me as a pitiable person and started addressing me again in person instead of asking my wife what I wanted.

In order to keep my head above water in these difficult, melancholic times of my injured life, I went looking for valuable insights into the darkest of feelings. A better understanding of depression should keep that feeling manageable (especially when supported by my mental resilience reflex) and stop it from sprouting deep, compulsive roots in my recovering brain. Whenever it got a hold of me, it was particularly hard to interact with others and to engage in meaningful work – things that under normal circumstances went pretty well by now. The long struggle had armed me well against the darkness of my mind, but the difficulty of the situation was often too great to be warded off completely. I came across a definition of depression as 'a lack of being'. That I knew all too well: the feeling of ceasing to exist and relapse attempting to take deeper roots. Luckily, I was determined to keep gradually building up and I refused to be shut down by negative feelings. I had to keep moving, covering distances, establishing connections, especially because it was feelings of social alienation and seclusion that were most dominant. In spite of the strong and beautiful people supporting me, at times, the connections didn't cut it for me. Luckily, there were ways of breaking free from my isolation, although it required a lot of energy and continuous exertion. I wanted nothing more than to belong again and that aspiration became an ever more important project of my recovery.

Therefore, over the next couple of weeks I returned to work for the third time in my recovery. From March to June, I would build up from four to six, eight and ultimately to 10 hours. The prospect alone already gave me a lot of energy. I felt so motivated. Throughout the first week of the six-hour schedule, I often noticed that taking things slowly was still a necessity. Classes with overactive students confronted me with my diminished load capacity and it took all of my endurance to make it through the first week successfully. Efficiently and correctly orienting myself in time also remained difficult. I often experienced irrational time pressure and felt stressed because of it. This posed a major challenge to the resumption of my work and life and thus it required a lot of deliberation and corrective action. I tried to use my awareness of the hurdles ahead to progress, to 'keep calm and carry on'. I pulled it off, but it became clear that although I still loved teaching, it nonetheless took a lot of effort and required a rational approach free from any unrealistic expectations.

The experience also demonstrated just how much I was alienated from society. This alienation seemed partly permanent. The distance between me and those I worked and lived with seemed strewn with the fragments of blown-up bridges. Despite my extraverted and open nature, I had a hard time establishing and maintaining a connection with others. There was a lot of uncertainty and my emotional housekeeping was often jeopardised by external challenges. I worked with a couple of new classes that were made up of a lot of vulnerable girls with ASD. This meant they often had to be excused because of emotional pressure and seek the help of the paramedical team. My empathy came naturally and didn't require any effort: it was as if we were living through the same circumstances together. I took it upon myself to tackle the alienation from society people with ASD often experience. I thought of ways to create social cohesion from the perspective of someone with an ABI – yet another ambition that sprang from necessity. As such, my philosophy classes once again were revised. I tried to make sure my professional approach prevailed, for which I really needed the support of my colleagues. Luckily, Campus Impuls – without exaggeration – truly was my second home. We worked as a team, even now in the case of my vulnerability. I felt an enormous urge to be a part of this again, but it would be a tough challenge, certainly not less so than all the previous ones, and it would take many years to fully reintegrate. My family and work had become my main focus for a valuable continuation of my life, now more than ever.

Here too it seemed hard to rein in my brain. I wanted to develop a new method with my colleagues to optimise collaboration. I proposed to them and to the board to use philosophy teachers as an extension of the care team, not by default every single day, but when the situation called for it. I also added that I wanted it to be part of my recovery on the work floor. I wanted to be involved and invest energy in it. It soon became clear that my colleagues were already in the process of improving care in our pedagogical project, so I saw the opportunity to contribute more to these operations in the near future. Initially, though, I wanted to focus on the classes themselves and aspired to teach my pupils the fundamentals of thinking 'carefully' (i.e. critically) in order to improve their resistance against extreme ideologies and nonsense in general.

In spring, I managed to partake in yet another event that would improve my integration. My band, 'Les Cochons Sublimes', was given the opportunity to perform at a music pub called 'The Crossover' in Ghent, a venue that invested a lot in sound and stage. I did everything I could to be a part of it, and I succeeded. The place was full and many people were aware of my situation. We were given a warm welcome and the feedback afterwards was positive. I felt the energy rush through my body. For days, I reminisced about the experience. As I said to the public during the performance: 'ladies and gentlemen, as you can see, we do it because we can and because we love doing it.' Also, I had asked Bart, the director of the documentary on facial surgery, whether he was willing to shoot the entire concert to make a concert movie out of it. It was a unique opportunity and I didn't want to let it slip away. Bart agreed and both he and his daughter Mariska were present with their cameras.

A number of meetings, either random (Maarten and Ignaas) or premeditated (Jan in a coffee bar, Johan online, Stine, former classmates Katrien Devolder and Ico Maly), contributed to this. I met Katrien at a philosophical festival, where she addressed contemporary dilemmas caused by technological progress (such as self-driving cars) as a moral philosopher studying applied ethics. Again I met with someone from the 'distant' past as a confirmation of my continued existence. I used the occasion to strike up a conversation, as I did more and more often those days, looking to establish 'opportunistic research communities' to test my views on reality. It seemed like I derived this ability from my professional experience with the Socratic method. Connecting in this manner broke the wall of my social isolation, fought off feelings of loneliness and improved my reintegration. The diminished sense of restraint the brain injury had left me with was – much to my satisfaction – of great help: I wanted to make the most of this altered trait of my personality.

And then, of course, there was the positive and (deliberately) optimistic interaction with my two daughters! I celebrated our valuable connection by enthusiastically partaking in whatever it was they did: doing homework, playing in the house and in the garden, enjoying their hobbies, having fun, being silly … It helped to breathe new life into my faltering trajectory. Intuitively, the horizon seemed once again within reach and I renewed the efforts made so far. Floor and Sien contributed most to giving my life new hope for a beautiful destination and remained my most important source of motivation.

Still, all these exciting personal victories didn't come easy. The permanent and chronic nature of my impairments had a big impact on the course of my emotional life. I felt forced to resort more often and with more awareness to the ultimate light in the darkness: my mental resilience reflex. Increasingly running or teaching alone didn't suffice to achieve physical relaxation or cognitive balance, and the days I wasted away ruminating to no satisfactory conclusion grew in number. After some reflection, I assumed the reason was to be found in the aftershocks of the many relapses in the past couple of years and in the relentless fatigue I was still struggling with. Oftentimes, I didn't sleep for more than three to four hours – a well-known trait of brain injury. The situation, moreover, was made worse by the endless cascade of thoughts in my head that kept me up at night.

My brain, in spite of its relentless stream of thoughts, still managed to make focussed efforts. There was a continuous flow of new ideas and unexploited opportunities for reflection, allowing me to not only think about my situation all the time, but to use my restlessness for other purposes as well. And so, in the spring of 2019, one month before the second anniversary of my recovery, I started working on a new project regarding one aspect of the operations at Campus Impuls.

> Our school assists (sometimes fragile) youngsters with ASD. Our central mission is to offer knowledge and to stimulate the cognitive development of our pupils. But there is more. It is also our duty to provide emotional rest and wellbeing. Our paramedical team spearheads this operation and also supports teachers on their mission. Along with physical education and social skills, the philosophy teaching group could become the extension of the paramedical team, positioning ourselves between care and knowledge transfer. This fits nicely our school's ambition of establishing extracurricular 'time-out programmes' on campus.

In consultation with my colleagues, I started writing a vision statement of the relationship between the educational and the pedagogical side of our operations. My thoughts were unstoppable, so I had to make the most of them. Still, it often made me wonder whether I would continue to use my reaction to these extreme circumstances as a benchmark for appreciating life. This to me seemed an unpleasant prospect: remaining this much in fighting mode would be quite tiring. The fighting mode had served me well during recovery, but I had to be careful that it wouldn't thwart experiencing the happiness of the here and now. We lose happiness when we believe it to be elsewhere, so besides my hunger for the future, I also had to be content with what I had achieved so far, to learn how to cherish these concrete accomplishments. To laugh and to fight would be a difficult combination. Would I ever truly be able to look back on all this as a permanently finished chapter? The idea of it was both comforting and strange at the same time. I wanted to be happy and optimistic, to enjoy my 'second life', so I decided to keep counting my blessings of everyday happiness and to cherish the present as a well-deserved bonus: I am, therefore I validate.

At the time, I also increased my running distance to a steady 10 km, sometimes even more than that, but hardly ever less. At the symbolic end of two years of recovery, I still felt the progress I could make. It was a true mental boost. Nonetheless, I once again ran into the contradictory nature of my recovery. On the one hand, I succeeded at preserving constructive levers for my mental balance and even at augmenting their number. Besides long-distance running, I now also spent the days working on four texts: a contribution to a manuscript called 'De kunst van Dirk De Keyzer'[1] ('The Art of Dirk De Keyzer', yet to be published), Book 1 (the one you are reading now) and 2 (yet to be published) and the vision statement called 'De les levensbeschouwing – tussen zorg en kennisoverdracht' ('Philosophy Courses – Between Care and Knowledge Transfer'). Forcing myself to do so, however, was still very much a necessity, because the fatigue and the daily struggle for reintegration took their toll. The passing of time and the upcoming second anniversary of the accident gave rise to an unprecedented form of persisting melancholy. I often felt chronically vulnerable, impaired and radically changed against my will. The search for a new identity was a lengthy one, forcing me to deal with the melancholy of finiteness. How could I turn this emotion into an ally for life? I didn't want to make problems 'bigger than they had to be' and make others worry about me, because I had things under control. Fortunately, I still had the monthly consultations with the neuropsychologist at K7 to look forward to. The idea of more intensive follow-up care was slowly growing on me. Decent therapy by someone with a talent for professional empathy didn't sound that bad. I convinced myself to be at least open to the idea for the time being.

Besides my running speed, I also increased the intensity of my work resumption to 10 hours a week. The pressure was palpable, especially on my cycling trip to work. I had a hard time remaining calm and tolerant of other road users who to my mind were behaving irresponsibly – in particular cars who didn't give way to cyclists and pedestrians when they had to. I had to suppress my anger and often made irritated arm gestures. I realised that this of course was triggered by my history as a road traffic victim and it made me wonder whether riding my bike or walking during the morning rush hour would ever truly be an option again. I refused, however, to give in to these frightful feelings and became an overly careful cyclist. I may have looked like an excessively ornate and overconfident Christmas tree, but I persisted in claiming my freedom as a weak road user. I never would have guessed that daily routine would be so cumbersome, even before getting to the actual order of the day.

I shed tears of joy at the end of the first week with 10 hours of classes and two hours of class council (mid May 2019). I braved the storm and made it out in one piece. A couple of classes were wrapped up by Edwin (my replacement at the time) and Tim, the Roman Catholicism teacher. This in combination with the care and quality provided by my first replacement, Sofie, would turn out to be an added value both to us and to the pupils. It felt great to be part of such a solid team of philosophy teachers and to take this extra big step away from my confinement. The future was looking bright.

I attended a workshop by an organisation called 'Creatief Schrijven' ('Creative Writing') on independent book editing. I now was convinced that publishing a valuable and beautiful literary product was possible even without professional help. This was one more worry I could cross off my list and it gave me the confidence and peace of mind I needed. I would give the professional approach one more year: if by then it hadn't worked out, I would do it myself. After all the hurdles I had had to conquer so far, this one wouldn't stop me now. There would be an edition of my book, no matter what. It was simply too important for my recovery. Working on it was a way of reflecting on my life from a distance. Bart, the documentary director, proof-read part of it and told me I seemed to be using some kind of helicopter perspective. I did so to deal with reality, to create structure through my story, to channel my energy and to affirm in writing that even living a complicated life can be worth it.

Despite the meaningless triviality of what had happened to me, it was my desire for meaning that made my endeavours hopeful. My aspirations were not pie-in-the-sky and I intuitively understood that positive expectations should be rooted in realism (here, now, temporary and modest). In this too I had no other choice: it was either this or losing myself. A large part of my former self had been eradicated, but nonetheless, I clang to the conviction that life was worth living in an attempt to react bravely to the situation. Learning how to live with my manifest vulnerability and relying on the support of those around me were useful foundations for my hopeful reaction.

The struggle with my self-perception and the permanent changes in my personality forced me to work on expanding and changing the concepts that underpinned my thinking. All existing patterns of my perspective on life were wiped away and had to be redesigned from scratch. There was barely a mental framework, structure, category or 'thinking track' of my former self left. I was no longer free and unconcerned, but needed more structure instead, both in thinking and in the physical realm: all that was crooked had to be straightened. Reconstruction was unavoidable and consumed all available energy. The unexpected advantage that I tried to make the most of was, however, was that there was no longer a limit to my creativity. Every insight felt unanticipated and new.

At times, though, my attempts to create a new structure for my brain had their excesses. I had to keep myself from assigning spiritual value to the number 10, which played an important part in my recovery:

- I succeeded at teaching 10 hours of classes a day again.
- I often expressed the ambition among friends to remain care-free for the next 10 years.
- I wanted to reach my maximally attainable running distance 10 years after the accident by the age of 50.
- My wife reminded me that in 10 years' time, both of our children would be adults.

But most remarkably, my default distance for 'glorified speed-walking' was now a steady 10 km – 9,940 m, to be exact, starting from and ending at my doorstep. Only 60 m short! Most of the time I left it at that, because I knew those 60 m weren't going to make any significant difference in my physical recovery. Sometimes, however, I obliged my pattern-craving brain (it deserved a treat every now and again) by rounding up to an even 10 km via a small detour. In the end, I even noticed I took the outer edges of the bends on my route to make it an even number.

I realised that our brain loves to make connections – a trait with many evolutionary advantages, but also with its pitfalls. It made me prone to creating the wrong patterns. Of course the number 10 had no influence on my life, that connection only existed in my head. In a sense, it was a relief to see that my brain was still working, with all its upsides and downsides. Another thing I noticed was that under emotional circumstances, my brain was more open to these irrational yet comforting connections. I therefore allowed the number 10 to be a suiting embodiment of completed objectives, a nice even figure to use as a reassuring reference.

During the second week of my 10-hour workdays, my fragility and diminished load capacity were laid bare by a difficult incident. I had to set a boundary with a pupil and pointed out his socially undesirable behaviour – an important part of a teacher's job that, as I knew from experience, really could make a difference to these youngsters. I wanted to help him overcome his self-imposed impairment and develop his potential to the fullest. More concretely: the pupil refused to pay attention in class and worked on a project for his end terms instead. I showed understanding and respect by allowing it for the first part of class if we agreed on an end time, where after I would demand he participate again. I elaborately explained the reason for this limit and the reciprocal nature of respect and understanding. The pupil, however, simply proceeded to stand up and walk out of the room to go and work somewhere else. I followed up on the situation to nonetheless generate positive learning outcomes by using the principles of non-violent resistance.[2] Again I managed to get to the true essence of my job, this time under difficult circumstances. I was still very vulnerable, so I asked my colleagues whether there was any risk of aggression in the matter, just to make sure. Their negation was a much-needed reassurance, as the unrest I felt was a serious threat to my sleep and mental stability. Indeed, the pedagogical aspect of the job would remain a challenge for the rest of my career.

Luckily, the story had a happy ending: the pupil voluntarily restored contact (it only took a little nudge from me to motivate him to do so) and during our conversation, he made a strong case for their point of view. I, in turn, explained to him that offering valuable perspectives for the future is one of the most important objectives of a philosophy teacher and the essence of the course. He said he understood and I was pleasantly surprised by his argumentative abilities and his willingness to see things from my perspective – both valuable and profitable skills for the future. By setting a boundary without reproach and reacting constructively to a refusal to participate in class, I maintained personal contact and gave him the opportunity to make things right themselves.

Once again, I was confronted with the versatile nature of harsh reality. Making a difference clearly took its toll mentally. On the one hand, I often doubted my capacities as a teacher and needed all of my colleagues to reassure me in this matter. On the other hand, I realised time and time again that a worthy alternative for this line of work would be hard to find. This motivated me to carry on. I looked for ways to let go without crashing and worked on a new plan of approach at my 'headquarters' – the teachers' lounge. The objective was to be part of daily operations again and thus to reduce my sense of isolation. I used to joke to my colleagues that 'I was going to be daft somewhere else, but I wound up back here.' It was my way of making letting go of my former self easier. I also gave in to the irresistible urge to hand out coffee pods, which were much in demand among my colleagues and served as a way to justify my own need for coffee. I became a mood setter out of necessity and conviction …

And as far as being a mood setter was concerned, I had my eldest daughter as an example. She had organised her Spring Festival[3] almost completely on her own, taking charge of decorations, entertainment and the thank-you gifts for the guests, while her mum and I had only taken care of the tent and a speech for the formal part of the ceremony. Moreover, she had been the host of the school's ceremonies, smoothening the transitions between different episodes. At the time, I came to realise that this was what I had been fighting for all along: to be a part of this in a conscious and acceptable way. I was a member of the family again and it's hard to express in words how proud I was of my children. They had been so strong, living hopefully and caringly in the present, working on a valuable future. I was there. I saw it. Life went on and I was still on board.

Four days prior to the symbolic date of May 28, the anniversary of the accident, things started to accelerate. Everything coming together lifted my restlessness to new heights and I had to draw on all of my energy reserves to keep the situation under control. I noticed on a daily basis that all these additional efforts took a toll, even the positive ones that contributed much to the progress I so desired. I had to work hard to keep balance and distribute my energy amidst all the input I received: I got the first mail expressing interest in my manuscript, the book about the art of Dirk De Keyzer with my contribution in it would be discussed on May 28 for the first time, there were many family gatherings at the time, my work resumption involved a lot of discussion and organisation, I tried to arrange an opportunity for 'Les Cochons Sublimes' to perform at De Gentse Feesten (Ghent Festival) and at other venues as well … These were challenging times for my load capacity. I spent many hours lying awake at night, felt constantly exhausted and experienced irrational levels of time pressure. Once again, it became clear that the struggle with the impairments would last forever. I had no other choice but to accept that to live means to change – I change, therefore I am, as it were. This realisation made up much of the canvas of my conscious mind. My goal, however, was to determine the course of these changes as much as possible by working hard, training my thinking and identifying my emotions.

On the morning of Tuesday, May 28, 2019, I woke up even earlier than usual. At about 5 a.m., I eagerly anticipated the start of this remarkable day, the symbolic second anniversary of the radical twist of my life. There was much work to do, but I was determined to make the most of it. I started by setting the table and waking the kids. After breakfast, I sang some English classics with my youngest and extensively cuddled both of them. When my wife and kids left for work and school, I waved them goodbye for a long time from behind the window. On today's schedule: teaching four hours of philosophy classes and discussing my contribution to 'The Art of Dirk De Keyzer' with the owner of his main gallery. My optimism didn't fail me on this emotional morning. The weather was exceptionally changeable that day, but in between two drizzles, I made it to school safe, sound and dry. Somehow, it felt a lot like revenge.

The week after May 28, the meaningfulness of my new life was once again confirmed. At work, I was facing a difficult dilemma, where every choice seemed to entail undesirable consequences – a situation that every team of employees is probably familiar with. In this case, we had to choose whether one curriculum would be replaced by another. There were strong arguments in favour of substituting IT for sports sciences, but it also entailed that some teachers and pupils would have to change schools. I helped to calm down this very tense situation full of miscommunication and clashing emotions. Along with my colleagues, I went back and forth between departments and used two insights to defuse the situation. First, there clearly was a lot of emotionality and I suggested using these emotions as an ally in the search for an agreement and not as a cause for irrational interpretations of the situation. I combined this with the useful insight that it pays off to be as least reproachful in life as possible – a justified approach, as no one had bad intentions in this matter. By talking our way through the week, we came to an outcome that everyone deemed valuable. The fact that I had been able to contribute to this confirmed that two years after the radical change, I had managed to establish a new, meaningful foundation for the remainder of my life.

And then there was the capstone of this eventful period. Almost exactly two years after the accident, the transplanted nerve of the left muscle of mastication became active. Slowly but surely, the left half of my face became operational again, the chronic paralysis of my body was partly curtailed at last. Now it was time to plan intensive mime therapy to keep this momentum going. This happened two days after I got the green light from the Dutch publisher of this book – talking about a fortunate series of events! I felt liberated: it was going to be a beautiful summer …

Ambitions and Future Plans

Although I had escaped death many times by the skin of my teeth, I had hardly been thinking of my own finiteness. From time to time, however, it hit me that I now was in possession of experiences and emotions that directly originated from the confrontation with imminent death and that I was still alive to tell the tale. Finiteness and I had thoroughly collided into one another as I made my way to the front row of the overcrowded festival of life. I had felt her, our skins experiencing the dragging friction of our passage slowed down by the masses. The contact had been intense, lengthy and over the entirety of our bodies – and then we seemed to be headed in opposite directions. Battered and bruised, I had crowd-surfed to the stage while death went for a couple of tepid beers at the bar near the exit. I had gained a unique perspective on life and death, the latter of which didn't seem so foreign to me anymore.

I imagined that the experience would have a major role to play at the inevitable close of my life. At times, I was overwhelmed by the feeling that I couldn't live towards that moment blindly – for that, I knew the experience too well. It had been of less importance during my recovery, when I had been forced to focus on survival. Back then, the priorities had been physical recovery and the development of my mental resilience, consuming all of my available energy for 17 months. Things seemed about to change. Now that the facial surgery was over, I entered a new stage in my recovery: it was the first time in a long time that I didn't have to undergo any major medical interventions. My physical and mental recovery now had the space to manifest themselves more clearly and my resumption of normal life would henceforth be less interrupted. I was still 'right here, right now' – and how! I was surrounded by valuable people and fortunate circumstances. Now I needed to sort out my priorities and define them in a specific manner – of that, I had already experienced the benefits in the past.

> Which goals are top priority? To what extent will I be forced to part with my former self? How much can I still do on my own? What level of impairment will I have to live with? These are difficult questions for my diminished load capacity and my overexploited energy supply. I have been asking them since the first day I regained consciousness, but they've only become more compulsive over time and have been constantly on my mind throughout the restart of 'normal life'.

My emotions had gone through quite a hurricane. It still was difficult to try and keep my ambitions realistic and durable amidst the promising increase in possibilities and it required hard work on an accurate assessment of my situation. Progress so far had been positive and hopeful, now it was just a matter of not getting carried away by it. My experience with existential void and finiteness had honed my judgement in this respect and reminded me of how truly authentic the awareness of my existence was. I felt a sincere connection to the inherently human search for constructive and concrete meaning, balanced out by insights from reading and running.

My top priority was first and foremost to be a father again to my children and a husband to my wife – followed by going back to full-time employment and staying active as a musician in a way that would not endanger my commitment to my family, of course. I shared my new focus with just about anyone who would hear it. It was of the utmost importance that the distance between me and the kids was decreased and – ultimately – removed. I would drop all other activities if that is what it took to be able to pick them up from school again, to help them with their homework and hobbies, to have fun and play games together. I wanted to be part of the family team again and to support my wife in the daily management of our household. The challenge would be huge and demanding, that much was clear, and it would take reliance on my experience and willpower to maintain my focus. I had already overcome quite a lot of hurdles through determination, but this one wasn't any less ambitious than the ones so far. It would be a lengthy, continuous effort, especially for someone with an ABI and with a diminished load capacity, but failure simply wasn't an option. I had come too far to fail now and it felt to me as if the ultimate success of my recovery would be determined by the outcome of my reintegration into my family.

Everything else was put on hold for the time being. A tough decision that I immediately made in this respect was abdicating my presidency at the parent-teacher association of my children's school. My engagement had been important, but could no longer be guaranteed, given my lack of energy and focus. Volunteering for this organisation was no small thing and required a lot of effort. I had to step back, which felt like defeat. Luckily, those around me confirmed that it was a wise decision and encouraged me not to be too harsh on myself.

The accident hadn't killed me, so I felt encouraged to come out even stronger. The ultimate foundation of that drive – to offer my children a valuable perspective on life – grew bigger and bigger over time. I wanted them to realise that, in spite of his random and extreme adversity, their dad had proved there are valuable options in life, that life is worth living, even in challenging times. They deserved as much and, as young children, could use some workable willpower. My life would be complete if I could offer them as much under these circumstances: it would mean that I had made a real difference within realistic boundaries, where life truly mattered. The restlessness of my altered brain seemed mostly to be focussed on this particular objective, thus allowing me to carry on time after time when things got tough.

When the neurosurgeons wanted to install the shunt, I asked whether I would still be able to run marathons. The answer was: 'In theory, yes, but we don't know anyone who has done it.' These words kept lingering at the back of my mind ever since. To me, it sounded like a challenging ambition to pursue, a vision from the future, with headlines such as 'ABI patient runs marathon'. It was music to my only ear still functioning.

Maybe it's realistic to run a marathon at the age of 50 – exactly 10 years after the accident. Send in the press!

In sum, I have two major goals for the future: playing an active role in my family again and resuming work. All other things should be considered side issues. This is no easy feat, especially since these so-called side issues contribute a lot to my self-esteem: long-distance running, playing music, reading and writing, maintaining and building networks. It's a matter of making decisions and accepting the consequent uncontrollable implications and it will be so for the rest of my life. The ultimate extent and finality of these changes is hard to foresee. Assessing future circumstances to me is a matter of days at best. So many things – most of them unpredictable – are at play and make an assessment of the remainder of my recovery as accurate as a weather forecast within a fortnight. This of course is true for the lives of all people, but I also must realise I've wound up in extreme circumstances, a situation in which unexpected and random events have a much bigger impact than under normal conditions. Indeed, it is an unexpected and random event that has brought about this situation in the first place.

The sheer banality and the gigantic, unanticipated impact of this coincidental accident is literally and figuratively mind-blowing. It's an outlier in the way things normally go – one with major consequences. It was mostly people in my direct environment (not so much I) who tried to come up with explanations to make these events comprehensible in retrospect. Apparently, for many people, it's almost unbearable to regard such things as meaningless bad luck. To me, however, it is an illustration that important events in life seldomly follow a pre-set plan.

One thing I've never done is ask 'why me?' I know the question exists, but I see no point to it. It spares me irrational feelings of depression and persistent feelings of abandonment. I've met people in recovery who were completely overwhelmed by the why-question. It seems to be a major crack in one's neatly constructed world view, a brutal pulverisation of an intuitively perceived bigger plan or harmonious connection between man and nature. Luckily, I've managed to avoid that mental crash. Through rational analysis, I shake off the rare moments when my brain goes looking for reasons why: there is no deeper cause, intention or meaning to the accident. I just happened to be at the wrong time at the wrong place and ended up with the consequences of irresponsible behaviour. The perpetrator had been found guilty accordingly and that's all there is to it.

Anyway, the accident has had a disproportionately big impact on the totality of my life. It doesn't fit in with a long series of events, all with their own subtle influence on the course of my existence. On the contrary: it's a radical and irreversible peripeteia of reality in and by itself. I am subjected to the tyranny of fortune because of an unintentional and directionless incident. This single extreme fortuity largely determines the final level of recovery and the feasibility of returning to normal life. I want an average life without any remarkable excesses again. When people ask me how I'm doing, I would love to be able to say 'I'm fine, nothing special, just the same old same old.' That's what it's all about, according to me: life as a largely predictable and gradual trajectory, where 'no news is good news' and the absence of any major cares is essential proof of its true value. Of course there are irregularities, even in a life as paradisiacal as that, for better or for worse, but at least they are manageable and scalable – ups and downs within the boundaries of what is controllable, as it were. (Loosely based on Taleb's (2012) 'The Black Swan'.)[4]

Even if control in life is an illusion, then still it is a useful and essential one, as is belief in free will. One in a position such as mine may just as well claim the right to have a couple of illusions 'for private use', if only as weapons in the fight for optimism. As I said before, the term 'illusion' in this context no longer applies. Just like 'free will' needed to be rephrased as the 'specifically organised will', urgent semantic action is required here as well. Maybe I should refer to it as a pragmatic and self-fulfilling conception, some sort of interpretation efficiently shaping itself in relation to reality (again, inspired by Maarten Boudry). 'Control in life' then becomes 'a thoroughly rational assessment of how life can be impacted'.

Moreover, I kept believing in the opportunity to make a difference as an important aspect of a valuable life – but not like a megalomaniacal adventurer or a self-proclaimed doomsayer, an otherworldly, cold-blooded CEO or a narcissistic sun king would.

Making a difference to others is possible on an interpersonal level by showing realistic and genuinely empathic involvement.

I considered this simple 'tested expression' the head cornerstone of my restart in life. In my work as a teacher, I had already come to know its value in the past. A thorough application of this insight seemed of the essence for a meaningful future. I wanted to be 'powerfully present', not just as some sort of decoration in the background, but fulfilling a valuable function in my family, on the work floor and in a broader societal context.

I realised that my story could be an inspiration to others, especially because I'm just an ordinary guy who nonetheless had achieved significant things in life. This is not exclusively the privilege of the big names among famous writers, top athletes, astronauts or CEOs – although their stories are the ones that get the most attention. I could tell a success story of my own, featuring an average Joe as the protagonist, a simple schoolteacher who wound up in a dark 'Extremistan'[5] (cf. Taleb) by ill fortune. That – so I was told by a stranger at a music bar called 'The Crossover' – was what made my story unique and inspirational.

On the one hand, the workable aspects of any mental resilience reflex vary from person to person. On the other hand, however, mine also has universally applicable elements based on species-specific abilities shaped by natural selection. Realistic and pragmatic self-fulfilling optimism can truly be achieved by most people. It is difficult, but possible, as is governing one's interpretation of reality and its consequent emotions. As I stated before, I discovered this key insight of cognitive behavioural therapy through experience, independently of any theoretical background.

Millions of years of evolution and adaptation to our surroundings have moulded our reactions to reality. Through evolution, our brains have grown into a large and complex organ. It is this mechanism, fine-tuned throughout the ages, that makes us fit for the search for viability. Our brain, with its huge, flexible network of specialised modules, allows us to adapt tremendously well to changing circumstances. The 'blueprint' of the human brain – developed unintentionally yet necessarily in the manner it has – has a biologically universal structure. Despite the many variations that come with big complex entities, the cognitive abilities of all people are (broadly speaking) the same. Circumstances permitting, we humans can be very resilient.

Despite my brain injury, this still seems to be the case for me, so I want to make use of it as much as possible. It motivates me to support others in their search for a useful perspective on life and all the difficulties it often entails. This much is mostly possible for all, given the right conditions. Therefore, it also seems highly commendable to me to improve these conditions for as many people as possible. I want everyone to have the favourable context that has benefitted me so much. The way I want to contribute in that respect will be the subject of a second book. This ambition will determine many of my future choices and behaviour. Our welfare and scientific knowledge allow us to be ambitious on a global scale, as is illustrated by my own story. I would suggest we make the most of this potential. May my personal struggle with impairment, difficult situations and extreme, random adversity be a source of inspiration for me and others in pursuit of this objective.

Furthermore, I had been working for months on a second book while the first one was still waiting for a publisher. It seemed meaningful to offer others useful insights for difficult life situations, both through writing and through physical encounters.

Throughout my recovery, I have met professors with impressive specialisations. The ones with a human touch in their professional interaction, willing to free up time for a thorough discussion, made the biggest impression on me. Not only did they save my life with their technological and medical wonders, they also improved the results of my recovery by treating me as a person. They gave me my humanity back on a physical and especially on a mental level. Prof. Dr. Hubert Vermeersch and Prof. Dr. Philip Blondeel (in charge of the facial surgery), as well as Dr. Kristine Oostra, Dr. Engelien Lannoo (affiliated with the rehab centre) and Dr. Virginie Ninclaus (an excellent councillor and listener to my wife, who had saved my left eye and thus most of my sight) in particular went above and beyond the call of duty, as did many therapists who worked with me. They made a difference to me, in the here and now, in the small but authentic story of my life. They achieved big, valuable goals on a very human scale. I could dream again thanks to their efforts.

I started to entertain the idea of celebrating my new life with a small party. I would invite everyone over to the workshop of a good friend of mine, sculptor Dirk De Keyzer. In many ways, the work of facial surgeons was similar to that of Dirk, which had given rise to the idea of the party in the first place. Even the tools were similar! Given that both the surgeons and Dirk were at the top of their respective fields, it seemed to me like this would be an interesting get-together – and it was yet another concrete ambition in the restart of my life to look forward to.

In sum, I had the growing desire to surpass myself, to turn adversity into energy, to use the impairment as a source and impulse in the search for a future. I realised that in the face of the absurdity of my ordeal, I simply didn't have any other choice than to make it into something valuable. Pointless suffering was to be avoided at all costs. As to how exactly I should carry the load of this tragedy, there wasn't exactly a manual or blueprint. Still, I had come to know the human condition and its merciless nature through experience, and from now on, I would draw life lessons from my victory over suffering. I pursued these ambitions with vigour, hope and optimism, as I still do today …

Summary

Finally, at the end of this book, I want to list the key points of my mental resilience reflex again, so as to better recognise, remember and elaborate on them. Together, they constitute a toolbox for rational and effective optimism. I want to stress them, validate them, make them applicable – in short, I want to develop a method that makes the most of general human characteristics:

- to strictly set feasible priorities;
- to build up with care, to take small but steady steps, to carry on slowly but with determination: 'distance first, then pace';
- to make goals attainable and to reject illusions, to transform them into effective and pragmatic concepts;
- to respond to irrationality with peaceful resistance;
- to turn emotions into allies, especially the 'difficult' ones;
- to see relapse as an inherent aspect of life and recovery: defeat every now and again is unavoidable and acceptable;
- to deal with impairment pragmatically;
- to repeatedly express and confirm the ultimate core of my motivation: to offer those closest to me (my wife, my family, my friends, pupils and colleagues) a valuable perspective on life, even in hard times;
- to enjoy the positive sides of the 'here and now';
- to direct my willpower whenever possible;
- to recognise the controllable aspects of reality and to hold on to them;
- to plan (pleasant things);
- to pursue attachment and collaboration;

- to seek connection with people I trust or want to trust by talking a lot;
- to maintain and expand both 'old' and 'new' networks;
- to work on my reintegration and to fight off isolation;
- to hold as few grudges in life as possible: it only consumes energy and is often a misleading, irrational construct;
- to acknowledge demonstrable problems without making them bigger than they should be;
- to avoid time pressure and, if possible, to choose the path that comes with the most manageable balance of stimuli;
- to influence my perception and consequent emotions of serious events (unavoidable as they are) and to transform them as much as possible into something manageable;
- to fall back on effective levers and to refine them: running, reading, writing, playing and talking to wonderful people, music, ...
- to continue the resumption of meaningful work with determination;
- to fight and to laugh;
- to make a difference every day on a human level for others and to cherish their presence;
- to work on my balance and orientation, literally and figuratively;
- to use humour as a weapon against victimhood;
- to use language against the impairment: to transform valuable insights verbally into landmarks of careful thought;
- to realise that meaning in life comes with moments of sheer bad luck, coincidence and existential emptiness;
- to accept that seemingly conflicting observations and paradigms don't necessarily invalidate one another: differences of opinion are often productive and profitable;
- to deal with circumstances that can be dealt with: to work on my condition to increase the level of my recovery, which in turn increases the valuable aspects of my life;
- to trust that tackling problems is often difficult but possible, as is completing objectives. This is not only achievable for top athletes, big leaders, artists et cetera, but also for 'average' people, for 'normal' people. Mental resilience is inherent to all of us as a part of the psychological and neurological architecture of our brain. The extent to which it is expressed depends on one's circumstances and personality, the latter of which you can somewhat alter if you go about it wisely. It's feasible and relevant;
- to construct favourable circumstances and to validate them;
- to be aware of my abilities and to use them appropriately;
- to work on a balanced, rational, effective and pragmatic focus;

- to remove randomness as much as possible from my thoughts and reasoning;
- to pursue optimism that is vigorous, but not naive;
- to cover 'long' distances at a sound pace;
- to use favourable coincidences to do even greater things and to achieve a valuable existence;
- to see the enormous diversity and continuous change in life, and to embrace it;
- to recognise the many advantages of welfare and to cherish the value of wellbeing.

Notes

1 A Belgian sculptor and a band member of 'Les Cochons Sublimes'.
2 See note 24.
3 A Belgian secular equivalent of the Catholic sacrament of confirmation, marking the transition from childhood to adolescence. It is usually celebrated with a big family party and celebratory ceremonies at school.
4 Nassim Nicholas Taleb is a contemporary essayist and a former option trader who has written a 5-volume series on uncertainty, which *The Black Swan* is part of. In his work, he argues that Black Swans (i.e. outlier events) become more common in history due to the increasing complexity of society. Predictability of these outliers, however, is well-nigh impossible, in spite of our attempts to do so regardless. Instead, Taleb argues it would be better to build robustness, i.e. the resilience to deal with Black Swans when they occur and making optimal use of positive events (Taleb, 2012).
5 Taleb uses the term Mediocristan to describe a situation in which the value of an outlier is not big or disproportionate enough to significantly impact the total value of data points together: the heaviest person imaginable will not represent more than 0.6% of the aggregated mass of 1,000 randomly selected people. The richest person in the world, however, will vastly exceed the total monetary value of 1,000 randomly selected people. A situation like that he calls Extremistan (Taleb, 2012). See also note 28.

References

Boudry, Maarten (2015) *Illusies voor gevorderen: of waarom waarheid altijd beter is.* Antwerp: Polis.

Taleb, Nassim Nicholas (2012) *De Zwarte Zwaan: De impact van het hoogst onwaarschijnlijke.* Amsterdam: Nieuwezijds.

Afterword

Letting go of this text and considering it finished is a difficult challenge. Working away at these words has been an important part of my recovery for several months. What started as a report of my ordeal has gradually grown into a therapeutic aid to give expression to my 'mourning process'. My wife has shown exceptional patience and understanding during the many hours I spent behind the screen of my laptop. The working title has been 'Between Hope and Brain Injury' for a long time. To me, it is an affirmation that I still possess a working consciousness, that my brain is still a functional organ. This observation is incredibly reassuring and motivational. Moreover, to be able to put in words the emotional impact of my exceptional experience is of the utmost importance to me. I have to do it now, because in 10 years' time, I will no longer be able to accurately recall what it felt like, how I experienced it all. Ironically, this period that I largely went through unconsciously will be one of the best documented phases of my life. In addition to a documentary, there is now this book. It is my way of turning adversity into something useful, as part of what I consider to be a meaningful restart. I do it because I can. I can! Wow! The book has become a benchmark and a landmark, a structure for reinventing my life. I will soon start working on a sequel under the working title 'More Hope than Brain Injury'.

This work has become ambitious out of necessity. It constitutes, if you will, a 'letter of intent'. Although the story itself is in no way generalisable and every ABI comes with different degrees of quality of life, it is nonetheless an attempt to illustrate an often-stated though also an often-underestimated truth: that life can be worth living, even in circumstances that at the surface seem to imply otherwise. Our welfare and cognitive achievements allow us to live through extreme conditions all over the world. If we do it right, this can become attainable for more and more people. Our ever-accelerating scientific progress and

DOI: 10.4324/9781003205142-9

technological prowess provide new and fertile soil for universal human resilience. I want to reach out to people in largely hopeless situations: war victims, the chronically ill, the severely wounded, people facing serious mental challenges, to show that, oftentimes, there are still valuable opportunities in the darkest of moments. Of course, there are situations which are so dire that there is nothing but despair on the horizon. Different people and different conditions inevitably come with different limits to resilience. Still, this is the story of one such dire situation and it provides a genuine example of a life unhoped for yet truly worth living. It goes to show that a meaningful restart of a broken existence is not an easy achievement, but oftentimes not as far beyond our reach as it seems to be. Therefore, my approach tries to be more than just anecdotal or sentimental. My testimony is an attempt to offer a new, useful perspective on life and to bring down the walls of isolation people often face in times of hardship. It basically says: 'you are not alone, there is a deep sense of connection and solidarity, I recognise and share the burden of your situation.'

Five years later, August 2021, as this book is being published in English, I am still struggling with the permanent changes I've been through. My physical therapist has become a part of my immediate surroundings and isn't doing a bad job at all. Mood swings and stress have become the new normal, especially when I cannot rely on daily routine (e.g. on vacations, changes at home or at work, the COVID crisis) and I worry a lot about climate change, in spite of my ambition not to make problems bigger than they have to be. My non-violent resistance against science denial regarding climate change and vaccines has only grown. The scientific method is the only way of gaining reliable knowledge, which we need a lot of in light of the enormous challenges we are facing today. My story, I dare say, is an illustration of that. I organise this resistance both at work and in my private life, mindful not to overstep what is socially acceptable, which I have so far succeeded at. Still, I can only make a modest contribution to the necessary mentality shift if I act wisely and find peace for myself and my environment, if I can learn to let go of what is beyond my control. To this end, I will make use of neuropsychological therapy.

The court case has turned into a financial dispute between lawyers and insurance companies. The judge's verdict regarding the compensation turns out to be to a significant extent a personal assessment, possibly based on so-called 'indicative tables'. We're not out of the woods yet, but I feel capable enough both financially and verbally to uphold my rights via customary legal procedures, especially since the judge seems to act as a civil servant in service of some vague common good in this matter. The person who ran into me is of transatlantic descent and as such has left Europe. There has been no encounter. I am still as determined as before to go through life with as few grudges as possible, but the ambition now feels different somehow.

I often jokingly state that coffee is the only addiction I can still allow myself to have, so I make the most of it. However, that isn't completely true. The injury has made my focus more precise and restless than it used to be, at times even compulsive. I'm now also 'addicted' to running as far as possible at a slow pace, reading, writing, doing chores that I feel responsible for and 'me time' – albeit mostly spent by myself. Indeed, the injury has alienated me, I'm no stranger to chronic loneliness and gloom. Still, I want to respond to it constructively, making the most of unexpected advantages and enjoying life while I'm at it. In my experience, these dark feelings too will pass sooner or later and there always is a chance to start again, something to look forward to. It takes a lot of time and deliberation, but it is possible nonetheless. It's the home-made art of living that has tools at its disposal in every household and comes to full and astounding fruition when supported by welfare that invests in wellbeing.

I am still working part-time and it has proven to be an enormous boost for my mental wellbeing. As far as my glorified speed-walking is concerned, it has become actual running again and I can now cover a little more than 15 km. My ambition of one day running a marathon again is therefore still intact. After all, it's not illegal (nor harmful, for that matter) to dream rationally. However, what contributes most to my wellbeing is the fact that, in spite of the changes I have been through, our family is still standing. This is best exemplified by the fact that my adolescent daughters love spending time at home, singing and having fun every day. We should be proud of that.

I get the feeling that I am covering a lot of ground in the pursuit of my goals, which is the fortunate result of an interplay of different factors and circumstances. I want to acknowledge the importance of being surrounded by kind, talented, beautiful and caring people and the confirmation of one's faith in humanity they bring about. Thank you, Katty, thank you, Floor and Sien, thanks mum and dad, thank you all, friends, family, caretakers and colleagues!

Epilogue

> If we can save the lives of people with an insult to the brain, we owe it to them to make sure their saved life is worth living.
>
> (Cicerone, 2009)[1]

The problems people with acquired brain injury face are oftentimes being seriously underestimated and getting too little recognition. Survivors may experience dramatic changes in their physical, cognitive, social, relational, professional and financial functioning, which comes as an enormous loss to them. It demands adaptation to the new situation in order to learn to live with the impairments. This is a grieving process that takes time – a lot of time. Following a brain injury, this process has a complicated course that poses serious yet important challenges to healthcare professionals and caretakers. Rehabilitation must therefore not solely be about remedying impairments, but also about dealing with the psychological problems accompanying the adjustment process.

Although the consequences of ABI vary greatly from case to case, the chances of a successful adjustment process do not only depend on the nature and extent of the impairments, but also on the response of the survivor and the environment. This is called 'coping': the way in which one responds behaviourally, emotionally and cognitively to (stressful) circumstances that require adaptation. Different people have different coping styles and not every style works in each and every situation. After a brain injury, both emotion- and problem-focused coping strategies seem effective and evolve over time. Examples of emotion-focused coping are optimism, encouragement, admittance of grief and acceptance. Problem-focused coping, on the other hand, involves dealing with specific consequences of the ABI, such as fatigue, irritability, memory loss … Less helpful coping styles, by contrast, are, for example, over-optimism, denial, minimisation and avoidance.

DOI: 10.4324/9781003205142-10

Moreover, research shows that in the long term, it is especially the coping style that determines the quality of life after the injury, whereas the importance of the objective severity of the impairments decreases with time.

One of the principal challenges of a brain injury is its impact on personality and identity. We 'are our brain' and when our brain is injured, it touches the core of our existence, which is a very painful and confusing experience. The process of growing awareness and insight takes a long journey of falling and rising. It requires a transformation of one's identity and the willingness to accept change. It is the search for a new self, pieced together from the fragments of one's former self. Of utmost importance is the ability to self-reflect in order to gain insight into one's impairments after the injury. Many people with ABI, however, lack insight, especially in the beginning, which means they are insufficiently aware of its impact on their daily life. This results in unrealistic goals that delay and complicate the adjustment process.

People with ABI often have a greater need for structure and predictability. They experience an increased rigidity and have a hard time responding flexibly to change or sudden events. This is often a source of distress. Their emotional resilience has been compromised, which in turn complicates their adaptation process and necessitates professional help and support, especially at the end of rehabilitation. If they cannot pick up their former life and no longer meet their own expectations, it is a severe confrontation experienced as an existential threat. This growing awareness is often associated with intense emotional reactions, such as fear, denial and anger.

People have the potential to adapt to personal loss. Professional care can facilitate this and learn the person with ABI to deal with the problem of lost normality ('I am no longer the person I was before the injury'). Therapy cannot erase the effects of the brain injury and must therefore focus on coaching the patient to know and accept the loss. Stimulating this awareness, in turn, helps to create a new identity.

Cognitive behavioural therapy (CBT) may be useful in this respect to identify, understand and change thoughts and behaviour caused by stress and negative feelings. Expectations, demands and ideas are altered and new adaptive thinking styles and coping skills are developed, tested and applied. Acceptance and commitment therapy (ACT), in turn, focusses on the acceptance of the new situation and the choice for behaviour consistent with personal goals and values. This way, people can once again have the feeling of living a meaningful life with their impairments. Narrative therapy highlights the stories of people with ABI and the way they cope with it in their lives. New positive narratives with a focus on strengths are written, centralising the person rather than the impairment, so that people can come to terms with their injury and reconnect with their values in life. By externalising ('you are more than your brain injury'), one gradually gets in touch with oneself again.

Besides awareness and recognition of the impairments, it is of the utmost importance that feasible goals are set and realistic choices are made by drawing on remaining strengths and abilities. This requires willingness to change goals and choices in order to increase chances of feeling successful – paramount to the reconstruction of self-esteem and identity. Empowerment is key here. People are assisted in learning to exploit their strengths, to take control of their own lives and to make the right decisions, so they will feel in control again. This way, they can give themselves and their lives meaning again. Finding a new life compatible with former values while acknowledging positive aspects of one's situation enables personal growth and significance. New adaptive and positive meaning in life is thus consolidated and makes people with ABI feel like they are but at the beginning of a journey, rather than at the end of one. The ultimate goal is to live a meaningful and fulfilling life again, connected with one's social environment, appreciative of what one means to them and accepting of what is no longer possible.

Surviving after an ABI is a challenge Stijn has risen to wholeheartedly. In his book, he has demonstrated how a person can grow in strength, from the occurrence of the injury to the struggle with its aftermath. The confrontation with the fragility of life can yield a new dimension and perspective. Overcoming his ordeal has made him stronger: even the invincible can be vanquished.

Prof. Dr. Engelien Lannoo
Clinical Psychologist

Note

1 Cicerone, K. (2009) Foreword, in Wilson, B.A. et al., *Neuropsychological Rehabilitation: Theory, Models, Therapy and Outcomes*. Cambridge: Cambridge University Press.

Appendix 1: Bibliography of My Revalidation

Throughout my recovery, I organised my own supplementary neurotherapy. As soon as I was able to, I started listening to podcasts and later on also reading books. What follows is an overview of the insightful literature that has helped to resuscitate my brain (in no particular order).

- Van Hellemont, Gertjan (2017) Wanderland. Radio 1, https://radio1.be/podcast-wanderland.
- Braeckman, Johan (2017) *Valkuilen van ons denken: Een hoorcollege over de kracht van kritisch denken*. Gouderak: Home Academy.
- Verplaetse, Jan (2008) *Het morele instinct*. Amsterdam: Uitgevrij Nieuwezijds.
- Bruers, Stijn (2017) *Morele illusies: Waarom onze intuïties niet te vertrouwen zijn*. Antwerp: Houtekiet.
- Harari, Yuval Noah (2015) *Sapiens: Een kleine geschiedenis van de mensheid*. Amsterdam: Thomas Rap. (English version entitled *Sapiens: A Brief History of Humankind*.)
- Dawkins, Richard and Wong, Yan (2017) *Het verhaal van onze voorouder: Een pelgrimstocht naar de oorsprong van het leven*. Amsterdam: Nieuw Amsterdam. (English version entitled *The Ancestor's Tale: A Pilgrimage to the Dawn of Life*.)
- Boudry, Maarten (2015) *Illusies voor gevorderen: Of waarom waarheid altijd beter is*. Antwerp: Polis.
- Singer, Peter (2017) *Effectief Altruïsme: 1) Ontdek hoe je het meeste goed kunt doen in de wereld: 2) Doe het*. Rotterdam: Lemniscaat.(English version entitled *The Most Good You Can Do: How Effective Altruism is Changing Ideas about Living Ethically*.)
- Verplaetse, Jan (2010) *Zonder vrije wil: Een filosofisch essay over verantwoordelijkheid*. Amsterdam: Nieuwezijds.
- Maly, Ico (2018) *Nieuw rechts*. Antwerp: Epo.

- Maly, Ico (2018) *Hedendaagse antiverlichting*. Antwerp: Epo.
- Taleb, Nassim Nicholas (2012) *De Zwarte Zwaan: De impact van het hoogst onwaarschijnlijke.* Amsterdam: Nieuwezijds. (English version entitled *The Black Swan: The Impact of the Highly Improbable.*)
- Devisch, Ignaas (2016) *Rusteloosheid: Pleidooi voor een mateloos leven*. Amsterdam: De Bezige Bij.
- Dennet, Daniel C. (2017) *Van bacterie naar Bach en terug: De evolutie van de geest*. Amsterdam: Atlas Contact. (English version entitled *From Bacteria to Bach and Back*.)
- Crone, Eveline (2018) *Het puberende brein: Over de ontwikkeling van de hersenen in de unieke periode van de adolescentie.* Amsterdam: Prometheus. (English version entitled *The Adolescent Brain: Changes in Learning, Decision-making and Social Relations.*)
- Devisch, Ignaas and Van Bendegem, Jean Paul (2019) *Doordenken over dooddoeners: van 'het is wat het is' tot 'het is overal iets'*. Antwerp: Polis.
- Boudry, Maarten (2019) *Waarom de wereld niet naar de knoppen gaat*. Kalmthout: Pelckmans.
- *Filosofie Magazine.* https://www.filosofie.nl/magazine/.
- Vandermassen, Griet (2019) *Dames voor Darwin: Over feminisme en evolutietheorie.* Antwerp: Houtekiet.
- Greenblatt, Stephen (2011) *De zwenking: Hoe de wereld modern werd.* Amsterdam: De Bezige Bij. (English version entitled *The Swerve: How the World Became Modern.*)
- De Poortere, Pieter (2018) *Boerke kijkt kunst: 54 woordeloze grappen*. Gent: Nanuq.

Appendix 2: A Brief Sketch of Stijn's Time in Hospital and His Recovery after His Accident (by My Wife, Katty Knaepen)

May 28, 2017: The Experience

On this fateful night, at 05:30, the doorbell rings. I notice that Stijn isn't lying next to me in bed yet. I remember waking up a couple of times at night and thinking as I watched the clock: 'He isn't back yet. He told me he wouldn't be long because he has started to train for his upcoming marathon. He probably ran into someone he knows. After all, it's been a while since he last went out …' At this point, I am still unaware of the fact that this will be the last time I let things unfold with this level of calm, that there won't be any other night I will react with the same peace of mind as tonight.

I go downstairs and from the window I see two police officers standing outside. As I open the door, I feel like I'm in a movie. The officers want to come in before they tell me anything. The voice inside that says Stijn has died becomes louder and louder. I let them in and notice my mouth has become dry. The officers remain silent and ask me to sit down. Then they tell me a car has run into Stijn and that his situation is very critical, that I have to go with them to the ER of Ghent Hospital right away and that I have to call someone to stay with the children. My first thought is: who am I to call at this time of the night? I try different phone numbers and am taxied to Dirk's house by the police. No one's home. The police call on our neighbours and the wife immediately comes over. I leave with the police. The children are still asleep.

It's been almost half a year now and I can still picture the ride very clearly: me, staring through the window, trying to imagine what I was about to learn … I remember that the officers had trouble finding the way to the hospital and had to ask me for directions.

In the emergency room, I was led into a small room where I had to wait as Stijn was undergoing surgery. The two officers didn't want to leave me and stayed with me. There also was a social worker to support me. I had been there before, but then as a health professional. It was a weird experience to be on the receiving end this time. I remember trying to convince those around me that I was ok and that they were free to continue doing their job (they were doing their job, only I didn't realise it at the time). I was sitting there for God knows how long with those three people when my parents-in-law arrived, along with Joke, my brother, Pieter, … At last, Dr. Vandersteene, the neurosurgeon who had operated on Stijn, came in as well.

I still recall him sitting there and explaining the technical situation with great care, serenity and a moment of silence every now and again. What I took away from his explanation was that they had given my husband a fighting chance, and that all that was left for us to do was to wait for 72 hours to see if he would make it. He was still in critical condition.

We were then allowed to briefly visit Stijn in the intensive care unit. Joke said goodbye, gave me something to eat and drink and went home, because she had to host a birthday party for Drea.

If I think back to Stijn lying there, surrounded by all those machines and tubing systems … I will never get that image out of my mind. Unfortunately – though I didn't know it at the time – it was only one of many images yet to come. It would be the beginning of an arduous medical journey …

How Do You Tell a Child …

I arrived back home that same Sunday. Our children didn't know what was going on yet. How was I to tell them? What was I to tell them? Everything that had happened had been so confusing to them and I could see the fear in their eyes. Looking back, I think I went into survival mode. I had to keep my calm, keep this family together and allow my children to go on with their lives in the usual way. I've always been honest with my children, I had promised them as much, I would explain everything to them in a manner tailored to their age.

I told them that daddy had been in an accident and would have to stay in hospital for a long while, that they couldn't see daddy yet, but that we would do so as soon as we were allowed to. I remember that Floor immediately came up with the idea to write down the things they wanted me to say to him in a hand-decorated notebook. They took a group picture and everyone had to write a first message to dad straight away. This notebook was given a central place at home, in our daily routine and in the ICU, until the moment they could go and see their father.

May 28, 2017: The Facts

Stijn was hit by a drunk driver while on a bike path. He had lost consciousness after the collision and was taken to Ghent Hospital by a St. Lucas ambulance, where he was immediately operated upon by the neurosurgeon 'on call', who decided to give Stijn a fighting chance. Part of his skull was removed to lower the pressure on his brain and a temporary drainage system was put in place. He was also given a cervical collar to stabilise his broken neck. There were many more (though non-life-threatening) injuries, such as a broken sternum, a broken eye socket, a temporal bone fracture, wounds on his knees that required stitches, a left eye that wouldn't close …

After his first surgery, Stijn was taken to ICU 1 of Ghent Hospital, where he was to stay for 21 days. They told us the next 72 hours would be crucial and that his condition was still critical. He was kept in an artificial coma and it was still not clear whether he would wake up by himself after those three days.

June 1, 2017

This was the day the neurosurgeons decided to install a Halo vest. Stijn had become restless and the cervical collar was not enough to provide sufficient stability, so he was at risk of sustaining further injuries or even being paralysed. The options were either a Halo vest or a permanent fixation of his neck. We chose the former, because it would result in more flexibility after his recovery. He was to wear this device for months until the fracture had healed.

June 19, 2017

Stijn was discharged from ICU and moved to a department called 'Neuro High Care UZ Gent'. Once his condition required less attention, he would be transferred to the regular neurosurgical B-department.

June 23, 2017

Stijn had fallen from his bed in Neuro High Care and was put through immediate examinations. They noticed an accumulation of fluids in his ventricles and that his fall had loosened a bolt of the Halo vest, thus destabilising the construction. The doctors called an emergency meeting and expressed their concern about an imminent loss of brain functions. They decided to install a shunt (a permanent drainage system in the brains) and to use a new, custom Halo vest. This was Stijn's second round of high-risk surgery.

Because of his unrest and confusion and in an attempt to avoid any further damage, it was decided to keep Stijn fixed on his bed or a five-legged chair whenever he was alone. He was kept in isolation in a separate room because of the hospital bug he had contracted. Stijn was fixed day and night, from that day until mid-September, for a grand total of three months.

July 10, 2017

Stijn's left eyelid was kept closed with temporary stitches to prevent dehydration – an intervention that unfortunately couldn't prevent his discharge from Ghent Hospital. He would have to travel from Ostend to Ghent for future consultations and to rely on us and healthcare service BZIO for daily care.

July 11, 2017

The day of the discharge from Ghent Hospital and the transfer to BZIO rehabilitation centre in Ostend. Stijn had run out of bed-days. There were no further medical interventions required and there were no vacancies at rehabilitation centre K7 at Ghent Hospital before mid-August, so BZIO was an unavoidable but temporary solution. In the meantime, we managed to make a reservation at K7 for August.

After a period of three weeks, the feeding tubes were removed from Stijn's nose and it was now up to him to eat and drink all by himself. This was visibly an exhausting and arduous trial, and he kept on losing weight.

July 11 to 17, 2017

Stijn was transferred to BZIO and had his first morning of therapy. It proved to be too much and they had to take him back to bed: he was too weakened and his consciousness was waning to minimal levels. He stayed in bed for a week, eating only protein-rich pudding and thickened water to eliminate any choking hazard. The weight loss continued and his muscles became spastic.

July 17 to 24, 2017

At our repeated insistence, Stijn was taken into emergency care at St. John's Hospital in Ostend on July 17, 2017. Given the critical condition he was in, they had to install a PEG tube that very same day. This was his third high-risk intervention. He stayed here for a week (the maximum number of available bed-days for his situation) so they could monitor the effects of the PEG tube. He barely responded at this point. His decreased level of consciousness led to a medical examination that revealed yet another neurological complication: sinking skin flap syndrome. Though in itself not life-threatening (yet), the problem required immediate attention. We had multiple phone calls with Ghent Hospital in an attempt to have Stijn transferred again, but all were in vain, so we desperately tried to keep him at St. John's as the second-best option. Again, we were told that his bed-days had expired and that Stijn had to go back to BZIO, along with a PEG tube and clear instructions.

July 24 to 25, 2017

Stijn went back to BZIO, where he had trouble breathing the very first night and was still stuck in a state of unconsciousness. The next morning, his condition motivated the doctor to call an ambulance for a transfer to the nearest ICU. We received a phone call from St. John's with the question whether we still wanted them to intubate Stijn and whether he had an advance directive.

July 26 to August 15, 2017

Stijn was back at the ICU, suffering from double pneumonia and a superbug infection. His bone flap, which had been removed because of the sinking skin flap syndrome, had to be replaced prematurely for him to regain consciousness. This posed three dilemmas: his Halo vest had to be removed prematurely, his bone flap had to be replaced prematurely and all these interventions had to be done in spite of the hospital bug and the double pneumonia. After thorough discussion with the professors and our family, the Halo vest was removed on August 2 and replaced once again by a cervical collar. They also performed additional examinations for possible infections of the four wounds caused by the connections of the vest. Two days later on August 4, the doctors decided the odds were in our favour and successfully replaced the bone flap: the fourth high-risk intervention. All we could do now was wait and see whether his body would accept back the bone or reject it.

The replacement of the bone flap was to get Stijn's state of consciousness back to the way it was three weeks after the accident. It didn't. Other complications had surfaced. The shunt installed at the end of June had not been finely tuned and drained too much fluid, which had an impact on Stijn's consciousness. He was therefore kept head-down in an inclined position. On August 15, they managed to find the right settings for the shunt, which allowed Stijn to lie horizontally at first and later on to even sit upright.

A week after the surgery, Stijn was again transferred to Neuro High Care and subsequently to the neurosurgical B-department.

August 28 to November, 2017

It took a lot of waiting, but Stijn could finally embark on his journey of recovery as an inpatient at K7 of Ghent Hospital. His programme included physical therapy, logotherapy and occupational therapy.

On September 14, when the doctors were following up on complaints of diminished hearing, they discovered brain fluids in his ear canal. After thorough discussion and examination, they decided to refrain from performing surgery because the risk was too high.

At the end of September, the PEG tube was removed. In October, Stijn started to swim in physical therapy.

On October 4, the cervical collar was finally removed and a softer version took its place for two more weeks.

Mid October

Stijn starts running through the corridors of K7 for the first time.

At the end of October, Stijn came back home for the weekend with his wheelchair and his walker.

December 8, 2017

From this point forward, Stijn would continue his recovery as an outpatient. At last, he was back home and went to therapy at K7 four afternoons a week.

March 26 to 27, 2017

Stijn was hospitalised at Ghent Hospital for urethroplasty as a result of the accident.

July 4 to 5, 2018

A sudden epileptic seizure at home landed Stijn in Ghent Hospital again. They prescribed medication and the suspension of his driving licence was renewed for six months.

September 3, 2018

The beginning of Stijn's 'continued recovery on the work floor'. Stijn is teaching again, four hours a week.

September 25 to October 2, 2018

The day of Stijn's facial surgery had arrived, a complicated collaboration between the plastic surgery department and the head and neck surgery team. A nerve from his left leg was transplanted in his face as the left-sided facial paralysis had not subsided and was there to stay. They also took some fat tissue from his left upper leg to fill the clearly visible 'crater' in his head, caused by the removal of the bone flap. In all, the surgery took 11 hours.

Appendix 3: Court Testimony (October 11, 2018)

I regret a post-surgical consultation with Prof. H. Vermeersch at Ghent Hospital prevents me from being present here in court today. On September 26, 2018, I underwent facial surgery in an attempt to correct some of the disfigurements caused by the accident.

In the past year and four months, I was put through eight serious medical interventions, four of which in life-threatening circumstances. My bone flap was removed and later replaced. I was given a brain shunt and a Halo vest had to be installed twice. I was intubated because of critical weight loss.

During urethroplasty and corrective facial surgery, my condition was no longer critical. Nonetheless, these interventions represent a major setback in my recovery.

The permanent outcomes are:

- a life-long acquired brain injury (ABI);
- a complete loss of hearing and balance on my left side;
- a disfigured face, mitigated to certain extent by corrective facial surgery;
- an unclosable left eye-lid, loss of my right eye socket;
- a decrease in my personal load capacity and a daily struggle with fatigue;
- a great loss of physical strength and stamina;
- concentration issues and a reduced short-term memory;
- tinnitus in my left ear;
- epilepsy;
- a continuous fight for mental resilience;
- a fragile neck after fracture;
- incapacity for work.

Through so-called ‘continued recovery on the work floor’, I am trying to pick up the threads of my working life, though the success of this endeavour is far from certain and considered doubtful to say the least.

My family, parents and immediate environment had to live with uncertainty about my chances of survival for months and were forced to a great extent to put a halt to their normal daily lives. My children (nine and eleven years old) have witnessed traumatic experiences.

Index

Locators in *italic* refer to figures

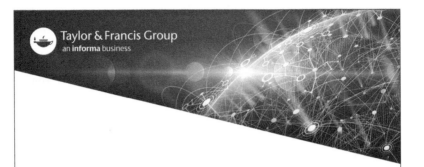